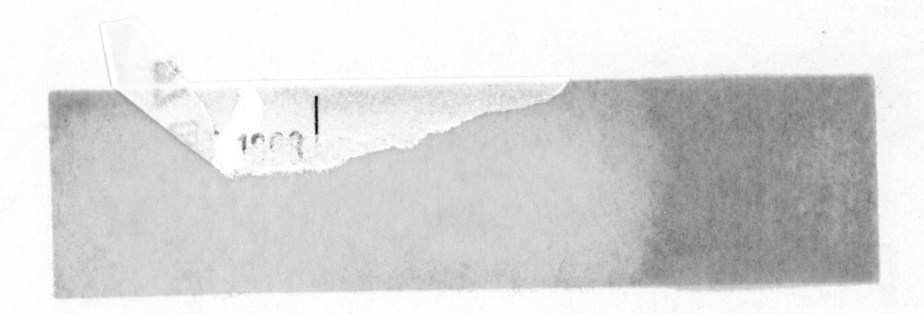

D1331886
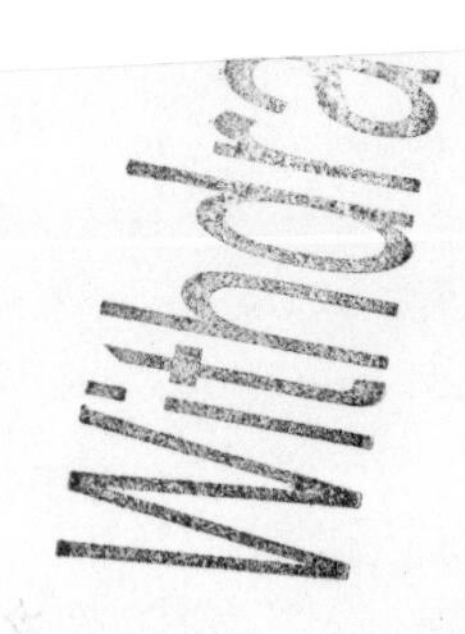

Professional Discipline in Nursing, Midwifery and Health Visiting

Professional Discipline in Nursing, Midwifery and Health Visiting

Third Edition

Including a Treatise on Professional Regulation

Reg Pyne
OBE, RN, FIMgt
Formerly Director for Professional Conduct and Assistant Registrar for Standards and Ethics, United Kingdom Central Council for Nursing, Midwifery and Health Visiting

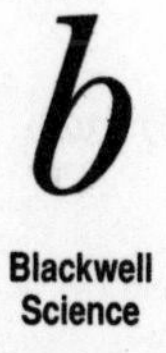

Blackwell Science

Editorial Offices:
Osney Mead, Oxford OX2 0EL
25 John Street, London WC1N 2BL
23 Ainslie Place, Edinburgh EH3 6AJ
350 Main Street, Malden
MA 02148 5018, USA
54 University Street, Carlton
Victoria 3053, Australia

Other Editorial Offices:

Blackwell Wissenschafts-Verlag GmbH
Kurfürstendamm 57
10707 Berlin, Germany

Blackwell Science KK
MG Kodenmacho Building
7-10 Kodenmacho Nihombashi
Chuo-ku, Tokyo 104, Japan

First Edition published 1981
Second Edition published 1992
Reprinted 1994
Third edition published 1998

Set in 10/12pt Ehrhardt
by DP Photosetting, Aylesbury, Bucks
Printed and bound in Great Britain by
MPG Books Ltd, Bodmin, Cornwall

DISTRIBUTORS

Marston Book Services Ltd
PO Box 269
Abingdon
Oxon OX14 4YN
(*Orders:* Tel: 01235 465500
Fax: 01235 465555)

USA
Blackwell Science, Inc.
Commerce Place
350 Main Street
Malden, MA 02148 5018
(*Orders:* Tel: 800 759 6102
617 388 8250
Fax: 617 388 8255)

Canada
Copp Clark Professional
200 Adelaide Street West, 3rd Floor
Toronto, Ontario M5H 1W7
(*Orders:* Tel: 416 597-1616
800 815 9417
Fax: 416 597 1617)

Australia
Blackwell Science Pty Ltd
54 University Street
Carlton, Victoria 3053
(*Orders:* Tel: 03 9347 0300
Fax: 03 9347 5001)

A catalogue record for this title is available from the British Library

ISBN 0-632-04086-6

Library of Congress
Cataloging-in-Publication Data
Pyne, Reginald H.
Professional discipline in nursing, midwifery, and health visiting: including a treatise on professional regulation/Reg Pyne. — 3rd ed.
p. cm.
Includes bibliographical references and index.
ISBN 0-632-04086-6 (pbk.)
1. Nurses—Great Britain—Discipline.
2. Midwives—Great Britain—Discipline.
3. Visiting nurses—Great Britain—Discipline.
4. Nursing ethics—Great Britain. I. Title.
[DNLM: 1. Nursing—standards—
Great Britain. 2. Clinical Competence.
3. Ethics, Nursing. 4. Professional
Competence. 5. Quality Assurance, Health
Care. WY 16 P997pa 1997]
RT85.P96 1997
610.73'06'9—dc21
DNLM/DLC
for Library of Congress 97-23059
CIP

Dedication

To my former colleagues
Mark Darley, Pippa Gough,
Tariq Hussain, Hilary Jeffreys,
Margaret Wallace and
Jane Winship
who will understand my reason

Contents

Foreword

Dr Betty Kershaw
President, Royal College of Nursing

On 1 July 1983, the new United Kingdom Central Council for Nursing, Midwifery and Health Visiting (UKCC), on its first day of life as the definitive regulatory body for the professions named in its title, released the first edition of its *Code of Professional Conduct for the Nurse, Midwife and Health Visitor*. On the evening of 2 July 1983, Reg Pyne, the UKCC officer principally involved in its preparation (and the first ever to consider and discuss the Code) introduced it and discussed its contents at a meeting in Manchester I had arranged especially for this purpose in my role as the RCN Association of Nursing Education's Regional Representative. The meeting over, informal discussion with a number of nurse teachers and some of their students continued deep into the night. It was evident that Reg Pyne shared my concerns about the standards of professional practice, had the capacity to address them from a different base and perspective than my own, and that we could be effective allies in the same important cause.

In 1990, in response to my invitation, Reg wrote the introductory chapter for *Nursing Competence: A Guide to Professional Development*, which it was my privilege to edit. He used the opportunity to expound his considered views on the subject of 'professional responsibility'. A year later, that theme was again addressed in a more developed form in his Second Edition of *Professional Discipline in Nursing, Midwifery and Health Visiting*. Both through the body of that text, and the numerous case studies and ethical dilemmas it included, he provided information about the essence of 'profession' and the means by which the nursing, midwifery and health visiting professions in the UK are regulated, together with material for individual or group study.

Now six years later, and following a period of years which has seen the passage into law of relevant new legislation (The Nurses, Midwives and Health Visitors Act 1992), an increase in public awareness and expectations, as well as significant government activity to reduce the level of regulation or even to introduce measures in many areas of life to eliminate regulation, he has presented the Third Edition.

As with the previous editions, the author, having examined the concepts of profession and professional discipline, provides a number of chapters which are, in effect, guides to the professional regulatory system currently employed in the UK. Similarly, as with the earlier editions, he also presents a quantity of case studies based directly on UKCC Professional Conduct Committee cases heard during 1995–6, inviting readers to regard themselves as members of that Committee and consider the judgments they would have made if faced with the facts presented. These, together with the studies of factual ethical dilemmas in practice, provide valuable study material for practitioners at any stage of their professional lives. The question 'could this happen where you work?' is repeatedly posed as a challenge to the reader.

The Third Edition, however, enables the reader to step further into the territory of 'professional regulation and enhance their level of understanding. Noting the arguments offered by the proponents of deregulation, the author has inserted a new Chapter 2 to explain his view of the essential elements and core principles of professional regulation and to indicate why it is important. The presence of this chapter, which explains professional regulation more generally before going on to use the UK system as an example of professional regulation in operation will, I believe, add considerably to the value of this book and broaden its appeal.

Also of particular note are Chapters 11 and 12 which form Section IV *Views of Professional Regulation: A Personal View*. Reg Pyne uses these chapters to take a constructively critical look at our profession and its means of regulation. He draws upon his long experience as an officer at a very senior level of the profession's regulatory body, now supplemented by his post-retirement activities which include a consultancy role with the International Council of Nurses to examine professional regulation. He is uniquely placed to offer such a personal view.

This book is about protecting the public and serving its interests. It is also about the standards and ethics of professional practice. I recommend this text to all nurses, midwives and health visitors, wherever they work. It is an invaluable guide to professional accountability. I am delighted to have been allowed to contribute the Foreword to this book since I, and the nurses I represent, share with its author a sustained interest in these important things.

Preface

In 1980, in response to an invitation from Blackwell Scientific Publications, I wrote the first edition of this book, then with the title of *Professional Discipline in Nursing*. That edition, while containing some previously unrecorded history, was, to a large extent, a handbook to explain the professional disciplinary procedures by which registered nurses, if the subject of complaint alleging misconduct, could be called to account and judged. It was, in some respects, a strange time to be writing such a text. The Nurses, Midwives and Health Visitors Act of 1979 had been passed into law the previous year and, when Government Ministers decided to bring before Parliament the Order required to bring it fully into operation, the legislation and consequent procedures that I was to describe would be replaced. I was, however, persuaded to proceed because there was no other available text that addressed these issues.

Having written the first edition while waiting for the 1979 Act to come into operation, I joined the staff of the new 'shadow' United Kingdom Central Council for Nursing, Midwifery and Health Visiting (also described as the UKCC or the Council in this text) a year later as its Director for Professional Conduct. During the interim period until the new legislation became fully operative in July 1983 I also continued as Acting Registrar for the General Nursing Council for England and Wales, that being the largest of the nine bodies replaced by the UKCC. It was then my task to help breathe life into the new legislation as the new Council got to grips with its responsibilities.

Strangely, in 1991, when the second edition (this time with 'Midwifery and Health Visiting' added to the title, and with a subtitle describing it also as an exploration of professional accountability) was prepared and published, further amending legislation was being contemplated to address the defects and deficiencies by then identified through the operation of the 1979 Act. Looking back, I can see that I fairly shamelessly trailed my coat about the changes that I believed should be made to the law related to the regulation of my profession in the United Kingdom. Almost immediately after publication of that edition, I found myself in the position of being one of the UKCC's small team engaged in detailed discussion with Department of Health officials about the possible form and content of a new Parliamentary Bill directed to amending the 1979 Act. Out of this cooperative work eventually emerged the Nurses, Midwives and Health Visitors Act of 1992, which came fully into operation in April 1993. As I indicate in the text that follows, the major defects that I had identified were removed by the new legislation, but leaving intact the excellent foundation of the former Act. It has been a pleasure, in preparing this third edition, to identify and celebrate the improvements that resulted from that legislation, and to seek to illustrate the quality of the legislation now in place for the regulation of the nursing, midwifery and health visiting professions in the United Kingdom.

In preparing this text I have also benefited from the fact that, during 1996, I was contracted to work as a consultant for the International Council of Nurses in its project on professional regulation and have become more aware of the variety of regulatory systems that exist. In the previous two years I undertook shorter projects concerning professional regulation in Hungary and Romania. This experience has served to inform certain aspects of my work on this third edition.

Chapters 1, 3 (previously 2) and 4 survive from the previous edition, but with some significant new material introduced into the first two of these. I have interposed a new Chapter 2, the purpose of which is to provide material which focuses attention on the essential elements and core principles for a good and effective system of professional regulation. I regard this as an extremely important chapter, believing it to provide a basis for the construction of an effective regulatory system, whether or not in the health professions. I have been pleased to supplement this chapter with the new position statement on professional regulation prepared and published by the International Council of Nurses in 1997 (see Appendix 7).

Chapters 5, 7 and 8 describe the legislation as it now is since the passing into law of the 1992 Act, and the processes and procedures that now exist for the investigation of reports or complaints that might possibly lead to removal from the register. Once again a selection of case studies (Chapter 13) the majority of them new, related to the contents of Chapters 6 and 7 have been included. Reference to Appendices 2–6 inclusive should assist in considering these studies. The 'decisions' on the cases are found now at Appendix 1. Chapter 14 provides a set of studies, again predominantly new, which will enable the reader to explore aspects of accountability and some ethical dilemmas in professional practice. I am grateful to my friend and former UKCC colleague Sian Morris, now with Bird and Bird, Solicitors, for the majority of the studies in Chapter 14 and the related 'B' commentaries in Appendix 1.

As one of those who was in at the birth of the Nurses Welfare Service in 1972, who continues to regard it as an important adjunct to the regulatory process, and would like to see it thrive rather than just survive, I again include a chapter about it (Chapter 10). I sincerely hope that my repeated explanation of its role and functions, and my final sad comment, might stimulate improved understanding of its importance and enhanced support for its work.

Chapter 16 is the chapter (replacing the former Chapter 10) in which I gratefully explain the defects in the 1979 Act that have now been remedied.

Chapters 11 and 12 are chapters of a very different kind that I hope readers will find provoke serious thought and constructive discussion about the state of the nursing, midwifery and health visiting professions in 1997 and the need for regulation that is active, innovative and supportive of good professional practice. These chapters will, I hope, convey the passion I continue to feel about my profession and the importance of it being seen to be regulated in a manner that genuinely does serve the public interest. In effect, these chapters, together with Chapters 1, 2, 3, 5 and 6, can be seen as something of a treatise on professional regulation.

In summary, I am offering the reader a volume that is part treatise on professional regulation, part handbook on the UKCC's procedures, and part study manual on professional accountability, supplemented by a clarion call or two about related matters that I regard as very important. I hope that you will find interest, stimulation and challenge in its pages.

Reg Pyne
October 1997

Acknowledgements

I am pleased to have been invited to prepare a new edition of *Professional Discipline in Nursing* and am grateful to Blackwell Science, through the promptings of Lisa Field and, more recently, Griselda Campbell for urging me to complete the manuscript before the opportunities and pleasures of retirement from my salaried employment grasp me comprehensively. Sarah-Kate Powell also deserves and receives my gratitude for her practical advice and help in the latter stages of my work on the manuscript.

I believe the publication of this new edition to be timely, since it comes at a time when professional regulation is under attack in many parts of the world. It appears also in a year in which the International Council of Nurses, in response to those challenges, has restated its position on professional regulation, developed by new supportive text. It has been my privilege to assist with that work. Another reason why I regard this edition as timely is that the regulatory bodies in the United Kingdom are the subject of a review commissioned by the relevant Government departments. Recognising all of these circumstances, although the book continues to describe the United Kingdom's regulatory systems in some detail, I have endeavoured to broaden its relevance and impact, and to state more strongly than before, why I believe that professional regulation is so important. I do this throughout the text, but particularly by the inclusion of much new material, notably that found in Chapters 2, 11 and 12.

As with previous editions, I include, as appendices, a number of documents produced by the United Kingdom Central Council for Nursing, Midwifery and Health Visiting (UKCC). The fact that the Council welcomes the use of its publications in this way and does not impose copyright restrictions is a service to the profession, and, coincidentally, helps to draw them to the attention of a wider audience.

I acknowledge my gratitude to those of my former UKCC and National Board colleagues, and other friends of long standing in my profession, who have persuaded me that my passion for effective professional regulation means that I have useful things to say about the subject of this book and should continue to say it.

I am grateful to my former excellent colleague and continuing friend Sonja Wolfskehl for directing me to Professional Conduct Committee cases which, in summarised form, would provide valuable study and discussion material to supplement Chapter 7 and illustrate the procedures and processes it describes. I am also particularly grateful to another former colleague – Sian Morris, now a trainee solicitor with Bird and Bird, Solicitors, but one of my professional nurse colleagues for several years at the UKCC – for providing many of the fascinating studies set out in Chapter 14.

Last, but certainly not least, I acknowledge the practical assistance and general encouragement again received from my wife Maureen, enabling me to bring the task of preparing this text to a happy, and, I must now hope, effective conclusion.

The material in Appendixes 2, 3, 4, 5 and 6 is reproduced with the kind permission of the UKCC.

The material in Appendix 7 is reproduced with the kind permission of the ICN.

Section I

Introduction to Professional Regulation

Chapter 1

What is a Profession?

What is a profession? What does membership of a profession involve? What exactly is professional accountability? Can the separate yet substantially interlinked occupational groups called nurses, midwives and health visitors honestly claim to constitute professions? These questions are often posed by people with enquiring minds, many of them practitioners within these groups. The answers they receive are not always adequate. I believe that nursing, midwifery and health visiting can justly claim to constitute a profession or a linked set of professions for reasons that I trust will become clear as the pages of this book are turned.

As for the other questions, after a decade of employment in a post which required me to operate the system whereby the profession of nursing in England and Wales was to some extent regulated through the statutory body's disciplinary process, and much of another decade fulfilling a similar function in respect of nurses, midwives and health visitors in the United Kingdom, the latter period having involved me in the preparation of *The Code of Professional Conduct for the Nurse, Midwife and Health Visitor*, I hold to the conclusion that consideration of some negative aspects (e.g. professional misconduct, professional negligence, professional irresponsibility) often helps to provide clues to some satisfactory answers. Let me illustrate what I mean.

A young woman appeared before the Professional Conduct Committee only a year after she first registered following successful completion of her training programme. This followed her appearance in a magistrates court where she had pleaded guilty to the theft of drugs and unlawful possession of drugs. She had been dealt with sympathetically by the magistrates, being given a conditional discharge for 12 months. She was the epitome of the person you would never expect to see in this situation.

The story began some months earlier when this young woman returned from a holiday in sunny climes with some friends. It had apparently been one of those energetic holidays which leaves you, on your return, in need of another holiday to recover. She returned to her hospital work, looking visibly tired. On only her second day back she was approached by one of the hospital porters. He was well known for his friendly and jocular remarks to everybody, irrespective of status and position, so she was neither surprised or offended when he smilingly commented on her tired appearance. She simply explained that it was all the product of her good holiday which had left little time for sleep.

The friendly porter offered her a tablet which he said would 'pick her up'. Unwisely she accepted it. It was an amphetamine tablet. Some days later events took a more sinister turn. The nurse was again approached by the same man, but now the mood was not at all friendly!

He reminded her of the unprescribed tablet she had freely accepted from him. He reminded her that, as a qualified nurse, she knew better than to have done so and he could now get her into a great deal of trouble. He promised not to do so, however, provided she obtained more drugs for him from the ward on which she was working.

In a state of great anxiety and fear, she did exactly that for several days, obtaining tranquillisers and sedatives by forging prescriptions.

After several days she came to her senses and realised that each further such action simply pushed her deeper into trouble. She lived at home and enjoyed a good relationship with her mother. She told her mother exactly what was happening and asked her to go with her to the police and subsequently to her nurse manager. As a result of her confession the police were able to detain the porter and obtain convictions for numerous offences concerning obtaining and supplying a substantial range of drugs.

While the magistrates who heard the case saw the event as uncharacteristic and took a lenient view, the employers decided to dismiss her. There had been nothing in her previous record as a student nurse in the same location, or as a staff nurse to suggest that her conduct had been anything other than satisfactory, but she was guilty of a serious breach of trust and abuse of her professional position.

The Professional Conduct Committee now had to decide whether this offence and the nurse's retrospective view of it were such that members of the public, when at their most vulnerable, were safe in her hands.

This case says a number of things that might assist in providing answers to some of the questions in the opening paragraph of this chapter. It illustrates that nurses, midwives and health visitors are subject to the law of the land in the same way as all other citizens. It then goes further and illustrates that nurses, midwives and health visitors who offend in such a manner will also be the subject of consideration and judgment by certain of their professional peers who, acting on behalf of the profession as a whole, have to consider their appropriateness to continue as members of the profession with all its privileges and responsibilities. In this case, while in no way condoning the unwise, illegal and unprofessional actions of the nurse, the Committee took the view that it was uncharacteristic, that she had derived substantial lessons from the whole sad experience and that there seemed to be no prospect of any repetition of this or other unprofessional actions. The information received about her knowledge, skill and competence as a nurse was impressive. The Committee decided that her name should not be removed from the register for the misconduct proved in a public hearing, but that some words of caution and counsel would suffice.

The matters raised in that case may be taken a step further by consideration of another case.

One day a consultant anaesthetist whose work took him to the operating department of a small hospital only one day each week, when about to sign for the administration of a drug in the controlled drug register, observed some entries which purported to be his and spontaneously declared that somebody had been forging his signature.

In the course of the enquiry that ensued a theatre sister admitted that she had misappropriated two 100 mg ampoules of pethidine from the theatre stock and made fictitious and forged entries in the register to cover their removal. Possessed of her written admission, her professional managers dismissed her from employment and reported the matter to the police. The police decided not to prosecute because the monetary value of the drugs did not reach the arbitrary level they were imposing at the time, below which they would not prosecute for theft.

The nurse appealed against dismissal from employment. Her appeal was heard by three members of the district health authority who upheld her appeal and ordered her reinstatement on the basis that the police had not instituted criminal proceedings. Her admission had not been retracted.

Faced with this situation, and mindful of her own wider professional responsibilities, the senior nurse suspended the nurse on full salary, but also reported the case to the statutory body for investigation and judgment. In due course the nurse admitted the facts at a Professional Conduct Committee. Those facts were adjudged to be misconduct. After hearing of the nurse's previous record and what she had to offer in mitigation, the Committee determined to remove her name from the professional register.

This case also makes a number of useful points. It illustrates that an employer's decision about a person's employment status is purely incidental to the regulatory body's decision about his or her status as a registered nurse. The same would be true if the decision to uphold an appeal had been that of an industrial tribunal or employment appeal tribunal. Further to that, it illustrates that nurse managers, faced with a situation of that kind, have a judgment to make. They cannot simply abrogate their personal professional responsibility on the basis of a possibly arbitrary or unwise decision made by other people. It also indicates that the statutory bodies charged with the responsibility to determine, for the professions they regulate, what, in a particular set of circumstances, is misconduct in a professional sense are not dependent on the criminal courts to establish guilt. They can receive allegations direct and, having operated the procedures which the law prescribes, arrive at appropriate conclusions.

Let us consider just one more case before turning again to the original series of questions.

At the conclusion of a hearing in which the charge against him had been proved on the evidence of several witnesses and then been regarded as misconduct in a professional sense, a psychiatric unit charge nurse was removed from the register by the Professional Conduct Committee. The very professional charge against him was that of 'failing to give appropriate care to a patient in his charge' in a number of specified respects.

He subsequently exercised his right of appeal to the appeal court, as a result of which the case became the subject of review by two judges.

This third case is cited not because the presiding appeal judge and his fellow judge dismissed the appeal, but because in doing so they emphasised that their primary role in considering such a case was to examine the evidence as to fact that had been given and decide whether a reasonable group of people, assembled as the Professional Conduct Committee, faced with that evidence, could find the allegations proved to the required standard. That standard, like that applying in criminal courts, is that the Committee must be satisfied so that it is sure – satisfied beyond reasonable doubt. The judges, having determined that the evidence had established the facts, indicated that they saw it as no part of their role to question the decision of a specialist committee, composed primarily of practising nurses, who had resolved that the facts did constitute misconduct in a professional sense and that removal from the register was the appropriate judgment in the public interest.

So even the eminent judges who sit in the Royal Courts of Justice accept that the nursing, midwifery and health visiting professions, through the statutory framework established by Parliament, have been given the authority to regulate themselves in the public interest and therefore have to make their own decisions as to the kind of conduct that warrants removal from a practitioner of the right to practise.

Now let us look again at the questions that opened this chapter: What is a profession? What does membership of a profession involve? What is professional accountability? Can nursing, midwifery and health visiting honestly claim to be a profession or a group of related professions?

Dictionaries are an obvious source of definitions, but sadly, in respect of any attempt to grasp the concept of 'profession' they are far from adequate. The word is more often defined as relating to the vows of a religious community than to any specialist areas of employment. Similarly the word *professional* seems, in the way it is defined in dictionaries, to have more to do with participating in sport for gain than with membership of an occupational group composed of people who recognise and adhere to certain ethical standards. This is not to say, however, that a study of several dictionaries is a wasted exercise. The following phrases have been extracted from the definitions of the word *profession*:

> 'A calling requiring specialised knowledge and often long, intensive academic preparation.' (*Webster's New Collegiate Dictionary*, 1980)[1]
>
> 'A vocation in which a professed knowledge of some department of learning is used in its application to the affairs of others, or in the practice of an art founded upon it.' (*The Shorter Oxford English Dictionary*, 1973)[2]
>
> 'Occupation requiring training and intellectual abilities, practised so as to earn a living.' (*The Penguin English Dictionary*, 1965)[3]
>
> 'An employment, not mechanical, and requiring some degree of learning.' (*Chambers Twentieth Century Dictionary*, 1972)[4]
>
> 'An occupation, especially one that involves knowledge and training in a branch of advanced learning.' (*The Oxford Paperback Dictionary*, 1979)[5]

These definitions at least have the merit of containing some relevant words and phrases, such as *learning*, *knowledge*, *academic preparation*, *training* and *an art founded on knowledge*. If, like me, you still find them woefully inadequate as you seek to apply them to the art and science of nursing, midwifery and health visiting, I suggest you note that they would prove equally inadequate when applied to the other regulated health professions. One might expect that a study of the definitions of *professionalism* would prove helpful. It does not, because it constantly relates back to what (for my present purposes) are the inadequate or unsatisfactory definitions of *profession* set before you.

So where else can we turn for assistance as we attempt to grasp and understand the concept of *profession* and to provide criteria against which to measure those occupational groups called nurses, midwives and health visitors? There may be other sources to which we could turn but I offer my two preferred published statements. The first is (perhaps surprisingly) one that appeared in the 'Letters to the Editor' columns of the *Daily Telegraph* in 1978. The writer of the letter (J. Ralph Blanchfield) first commented on the tendency to misuse and abuse the word *profession* and the need to define it, and then continued:

'"Profession" cannot be defined in terms of any single characteristic. To justify the description, an occupational group must fulfil not some but all of the following criteria:

1. Its practice is based on a recognised body of learning.
2. It establishes an independent body for the collective pursuit of aims and objects related to these criteria.
3. Admission to corporate membership is based on strict standards of competence attested by examinations and assessed experience.
4. It recognises that its practice must be for the benefit of the public as well as that of its practitioners.
5. It recognises its responsibility to advance and extend the body of knowledge on which it is based.
6. It recognises its responsibility to concern itself with facilities, methods and provision for educating and training future entrants and for enhancing the knowledge of present practitioners.
7. It recognises the need for its members to conform to high standards of ethics and professional conduct set out in a published code with appropriate disciplinary procedures.'

Does this improve on the definitions drawn from a selection of dictionaries? I believe the answer is an unequivocal 'Yes'. Those dictionaries variously described the role as calling, vocation, occupation and employment. They also refer variously to the specialised knowledge, academic preparation, department of learning, training and knowledge on which it is based. In this respect they compare only with the first of the seven points in the Blanchfield definition. Ironically it is on this very point that some people argue that nursing is not a profession. Nursing (they say) cannot be regarded as a profession because it is based not on a body of knowledge of its own but that of the medical profession.

Whilst I readily accept that much of the role of the nurse (and, to a substantial degree, the midwife) is concerned with the administration of medicines and the provision of treatment prescribed by doctors, there is very much more to nursing, midwifery and health visiting than that. I have no doubt that many patients who received, from nurses and midwives, only the treatment prescribed by doctors would feel very aggrieved. The many other things that go to make nursing, midwifery and health visiting practice what it is are based on an existing and continually developing body of knowledge and practical skills which, while often (not always) applied as a complement to prescribed medical treatment and drugs, can stand and often do stand on their own. On this knowledge and these skills those who aspire to achieve qualifications as registered nurses, midwives or health visitors are examined and assessed. It is therefore my contention that the three linked professions of which I write do satisfy the first criterion of the Blanchfield definition.

What of the other criteria? The second, in the case of the United Kingdom, is clearly satisfied by the existence, as required by the Nurses, Midwives and Health Visitors Act 1979, of the statutory body called the United Kingdom Central Council for Nursing, Midwifery and Health Visiting (UKCC or the Council). That Act places upon the regulatory body which it has created not simply aims and objectives but the mandatory requirement that standards of training and professional conduct shall be established and improved. I explore the response to this challenge in a later chapter.

The third criterion is satisfied in several ways. As required by the Nurses, Midwives and Health Visitors Act 1979 (now amended by the 1992 Act of the same name), subordinate legislation (rules set out in statutory instruments), prepared by the UKCC, states the requirements to be satisfied and the competences to be achieved for admission to the register as a nurse, midwife or health visitor. The UKCC also prescribes the type, content and standard of training required. Applicants for admission to the register in the United Kingdom following initial training and registration in other countries (excluding those from the European Community covered by specialist directives who have freedom of movement within the Community) are subjected to individual evaluation.

The fourth criterion – recognition by an occupational group that its practice must be for the benefit of the public – has effectively been answered in law in the United Kingdom, even if not explicitly stated therein, since the first Midwives Act 1902 and the Nurses Registration Act 1919. It has become more overt through the wording of the Nurses, Midwives and Health Visitors Act 1979[6] and that of 1992 and is stated in bold and clear terms in documents prepared and issued by the new regulatory body established by that 1979 Act since it succeeded to the role of the replaced bodies, and took on a much wider regulatory role in July 1983. These have carried professional regulation into more constructive and positive territory.

It is probably true to say of the fifth criterion that, while always receiving some attention, this area had perhaps received less attention than it needed and deserved. This is no longer the case. The number of practitioners engaged in valid research is most impressive. The much larger number voluntarily engaging in work directed to identifying ways in which standards of care can be improved and then establishing the means of achieving the new standards is greater still. In both respects this is extremely encouraging.

As for criterion 6, both from the profession's statutory body (UKCC) through its statements of its expectations of practitioners on its register, and from those practitioners as they work out their individual ways of responding through their practice and in their various practice settings, comes a clear indication that this responsibility is understood and accepted.

The final criterion in the Blanchfield definition requires that an occupational group 'recognises the need for its members to conform to high standards of ethics and professional conduct set out in a published code with appropriate disciplinary procedures'. Nursing, midwifery and health visiting in the United Kingdom undoubtedly satisfy this requirement, as the remainder of this book asserts and Chapters 7 and 8 illustrate.

I will assert, then, that, measured against the most satisfactory definition of a profession that I have been able to find, nursing, midwifery and health visiting justify that description and title. That does not, however, mean that I believe that definition to be perfect. There is one particular respect in which I would dispute the wording to some degree, though recognising that the differences are more of a semantic nature than of principle. It relates to the fourth criterion in the list. For me, one of the hallmarks of a profession is that it accepts the onerous burden of regulating itself, but recognises that this is to be performed for the protection of the public and not the prestige of its members. Such an arrangement exists for nursing, midwifery and health visiting in the United Kingdom. It is something precious which the members of the profession must safeguard. My second preferred definition was found in the text of a speech made by Lord Benson (an accountant by profession) in the House of Lords on 8 July 1992. In the course of debate he offered the following as the defining criteria for a profession:

'The nine obligations to the public are these:

- First, the profession must be controlled by a governing body which in professional matters directs the behaviour of its members. For their part the members have a responsibility to subordinate their selfish private interests in favour of support for the governing body.
- Secondly, the governing body must set adequate standards of education as a condition of entry and thereafter ensure that students obtain an acceptable standard of professional competence. Training and education do not stop at qualification. They must continue throughout the member's professional life.
- Thirdly, the governing body must set the ethical rules and professional standards which are to be observed by the members. They should be higher than those established by the general law.
- Fourthly, the rules and standards enforced by the governing body should be designed for the benefit of the public and not for the private advantage of the members.
- Fifthly, the governing body must take disciplinary action, if necessary expulsion from membership should the rules and standards it lays down not be observed or should a member be guilty of bad professional work.
- Sixthly, work is often reserved to a profession by statute – not because it was for the advantage of the members but because, for the protection of the public, it should be carried out only by persons with the requisite training, standards and disciplines.
- Seventh, the governing body must satisfy itself that there is fair and open competition in the practice of the profession so that the public are not at risk of being exploited. It follows that members in practice must give information to the public about their experience, competence, capacity to do the work and the fees payable.
- Eighth, the members of the profession, whether in practice or in employment, must be independent in thought and outlook. They must be willing to speak their minds without fear or favour. They must not allow themselves to be put under the control or dominance of any person or organisation which could impair that independence.
- Ninth, in its specific field of learning a profession must give leadership to the public it serves.'

I am comfortable with that set of 'defining criteria' and believe that, as with those enunciated by Blanchfield, my profession measures up to them quite well.

I believe this also to be the case in respect of the many other countries in the world which have developed professional regulatory systems founded on five key elements. First, the existence of a register of the profession's members, able to be accessed by employers and the public and which, in effect, declares that the persons on the register are those from whom an appropriate standard of conduct and competence can be expected. Second, control of admission to that register through education and examination processes in that country, or the comprehensive evaluation of applicants whose original professional education was received in other countries. Third, the preparation and dissemination of advice, guidance and standards to make clear to practitioners what is expected of them. Fourth, the requirement that they maintain fitness for purpose as health care changes. Fifth, the authority and the means to remove practitioners from the register and thus prevent them from practising if the public interest so requires. These five elements of a professional regulatory system are all, I contend, essential, and must all be applied effectively by the regulatory body if the public interest is to be honoured.

I hope that I have satisfactorily answered two of the questions with which I opened this chapter – 'What is a profession?' and 'Can the occupational groups called nurses, midwives and health visitors claim to constitute professions?' What of the remaining two? One asks 'What does membership of a profession involve?' and the other 'What exactly is professional accountability?' On reflection I think that these questions identify two facets of the same point – that which will form the subject of Chapter 7. For now I content myself with simply stating in broad terms that any person on the Council's register – nurse, midwife or health visitor – irrespective of the post he or she holds, bears a personal professional accountability which cannot be avoided in four specific areas. These I believe to be:

(1) his or her own standards of care and the knowledge, skill, attitudes, values and qualities of observation on which they are based;
(2) his or her concern about the environment in which he or she has to practise;
(3) his or her responsibility to care for and about colleagues; and
(4) his or her acceptance of a role that includes participation in the teaching of others, be they patients, clients, students or junior colleagues.

To those registered nurses, midwives and health visitors who accept posts which have a managerial component falls that additional burden (shared, with enthusiasm I hope, by those with line management responsibility) of striving, at all times, to create, sustain and maintain a setting and approach which is dynamic, so that all nurses, midwives and health visitors (not only those in training) may grow and improve, and thus contribute to growth and improvement in others. This duty, like the four listed above, is concerned with the safety of patients and clients and the standards of care available for them now and in the future.

These then are, in my view, some of the key points to make in respect of those remaining questions. You may not necessarily agree with them. Whether you do or not at this stage, I suggest that you defer judgment until you have read Chapter 7. I respect your right then to come to different conclusions about those things that constitute professional accountability and illustrate what membership of a profession involves. If my conclusions do not appeal to you I suggest that you prepare a list of your own.

I have little doubt that if you do that it will lead you, as it has me, to the conclusion that the nursing, midwifery and health visiting profession, through each and every one of its members must come to a recognition of its collective responsibility for regulating itself. While a special and substantial part of that responsibility is laid by the law of the country in the United Kingdom on the United Kingdom Central Council for Nursing, Midwifery and Health Visiting (through its power in respect of individuals and institutions), the remaining part, and undoubtedly the largest part, must come from the self-discipline of the profession's members. Without that, no matter how we define their word *profession*, we shall not deserve that honoured title.

(Chapter 13 provides further case studies concerning Professional Conduct Committee work and relates to the contents of Chapter 8, for individual or group consideration.)

(Chapter 14 provides case studies concerning the exercise of accountability related to the contents of Chapter 7.)

References

1 *Webster's New Collegiate Dictionary*, Eighth Edition (1980). Springfield, Mass.: G. & C. Merriam Co. By permission. From *Webster's New Collegiate Dictionary* © 1980 by G. & C. Merriam Co., Publishers of the Merriam-Webster Dictionaries.
2 *The Shorter Oxford English Dictionary*, Third Edition (1973). Edited by C.T. Onions. Oxford: Oxford University Press. Excerpts reprinted by permission of Oxford University Press.
3 *The Penguin English Dictionary* (1969). Edited by G. N. Garmonsay & J. Simpson. Harmondsworth: Penguin Books. Reprinted by permission of Penguin Books.
4 *Chambers Twentieth Century Dictionary* (1972). Edited by A.M. Macdonald. Edinburgh & London: W. & R. Chambers Ltd.
5 *The Oxford Paperback Dictionary* (1969). Edited by J.M. Hawkins. Oxford: Oxford University Press. Excerpt reprinted by permission of Oxford University Press.
6 *Nurses, Midwives & Health Visitors Act 1979.* London: HMSO.

Chapter 2

Professional Regulation – Essential Elements and Core Principles

At the outset of this chapter I must declare myself as a passionate believer in and supporter of self-regulation for members of the various health professions. That sentiment similarly applies to other occupational groups which claim the title 'profession', on whose practitioners individual members of the public must depend, often at times of anxiety, dependence and vulnerability. That said, I must immediately add the rider that regulatory systems (where they exist) will only survive, and will only deserve to survive, if they are seen to be achieving their important objective of serving the public interest in a comprehensive manner.

I am on record as stating, when a senior employee of my profession's regulatory body in the United Kingdom, that:

> 'If any one of us (meaning regulatory bodies) does it badly – or appears to be self-serving and professionally precious or protective – or fails to use positively and constructively the legislation that we have – or fails to identify the deficiencies in that legislation and seek remedies – or fails to operate a system which is manifestly fair, efficient and accessible – we let down every professional regulatory body and endanger the principle of professional self-regulation. In doing so we also let down those other occupational groups who aspire to regulatory status. The essential components of professional regulation in our times must include constant reappraisal and constant striving for improvement.'[1]

I still adhere without reservation to that statement, because professional regulation is not for adornment; it is for application.

Having (in Chapter 1) cited in aid the defining criteria for a profession stated by Blanchfield and Benson respectively, I stated my belief that such professions needed professional regulatory systems which include five key elements. The reader deserves some elaboration of this statement.

The professional register

The purpose of the professional register must, surely, be to make it known, to any persons who need to know, exactly who are the registered practitioners in a particular profession. The register should, in effect, be a means of declaring that the persons whose names are included in it are those from whom members of the public, and employers who contract with them to provide a service, can have reasonable confidence that they will manifest an appropriate standard of both competence and conduct. In order to achieve this the register must be known to exist, must be constantly updated and must be accessible.

What a professional register is not intended to be is a bureaucratic device, the prime purpose of which is to inflate the importance of those whose names are included, while affording no assurances or protection to society at large.

In order that the professional register can satisfy the reasonable expectations that others have of it and have any significance, the other elements must also be in place.

Control of entry to the register

The professional register is a meaningless device unless inclusion in it is the result of appropriate education and training in an approved institution, at the end of which the individual has demonstrated possession of the appropriate knowledge and skill to be permitted to embark on a career as a professional practitioner.

In the case of the nursing, midwifery and health visiting professions in the United Kingdom, the substantial majority of initial entrants to the register maintained by the regulatory body (19 632 in 1995/96) were admitted following completion of approved programmes in educational institutions within the country approved for that purpose. There is substantial direct control over that part of the route to the register.

The second largest category of initial entrants (1999 in 1995/96) is of persons whose original education and training, and thus their original registration, was in a country outside the United Kingdom and which was not a member state of the European Union (to which certain professional Directives apply). In these cases, the application is subjected to a detailed individual evaluation, account being taken of both the original programme and the applicant's professional experience since their original registration. Where the application is not regarded as immediately acceptable for registration in the United Kingdom (approximately half of the total), the applicants are informed what is required of them in order to make them acceptable for registration.

The third and smallest category of initial entrants to the register (though increasing as a proportion of the whole whenever its state membership is enlarged) is of those whose original registration as a general nurse or midwife was in a member state of the European Union. In these cases 'Directives' apply which govern both the duration and content of programmes of preparation and provide some guarantee of standard in respect of what they describe as 'the general care nurse' and 'the midwife'. The number of initial entrants through this channel in 1995/96 was 816.

These are the means by which control of admission is achieved as part of the total regulatory process. Admission to the register cannot be achieved without successful passage through one of these channels.

Removal of the authority to practise

Just as the register becomes a meaningless device if appropriate control is not exerted over admission to it, so also it has no significance if the regulatory body has no power, and no procedures in place, whereby, in the public interest, it can remove or suspend a practitioner's registration and, by that means, prevent a person from practising in their profession. A substantial part of this book is devoted to a more detailed explanation of the current system in the United Kingdom for such measures to be taken. I simply emphasise at this point that this is an essential element of the regulatory process.

Advice, guidance and standards

If a regulatory body possesses the awesome power to remove a person from its professional register, and thus prevent her or him from practising in their chosen profession, it must surely be incumbent on that body to provide, for all those whose names are included in the register, some clear statement or explanation of what is expected of them. This is achieved in the United Kingdom by the Council's *Code of Professional Conduct for the Nurse, Midwife and Health Visitor.*[2] This short but immensely important text provides, for the individual practitioner, a template against which they can measure their own professional conduct, knowing that, should they be the subject of a complaint to the Council which calls into question their registration status, the Council will use it in exactly that way. It also has the benefit of providing for the public a clear indication of what it may expect of registered practitioners. The code, and other documents promoting standards and offering guidance, are addressed more fully in Chapter 7. Reference to them is made here to point up their collective importance as one of the key elements of professional regulation.

Maintaining fitness for purpose

It is essential that practitioners who achieve registration status at a particular point in time see that not as an end but as a beginning. From this point they must grow professionally and develop themselves. The public will be very badly served if they find themselves in the care of practitioners who have done nothing to maintain, and therefore even less to improve their knowledge, skill and general competence, contenting themselves with an approach to practice which is seriously outdated. The good professional practitioner will accept it as a matter of personal professional accountability to ensure that they remain fit for the purpose for which people engage their services. But the good professional regulatory system will also include some means of seeking to ensure that this is achieved. This also should be regarded as an essential element of an effective professional regulatory system.

These five essential elements of professional regulation must be supplemented, in order to ensure that they are appropriately applied, by constant reappraisal and constant striving for improvement.

The benefits of professional regulation

It is my contention that, provided that it contains what I argue are the essential elements, professional regulation of the nursing profession has something of benefit for all those who might be regarded as its stakeholders. That is to say that it should be seen as something that matters to governments, to employers of nurses, to practitioners themselves, and above all to members of the public who, at times in their life that are usually outside their control, depend on the attitudes, knowledge and skill of professional nurses, midwives and health visitors and their approach to professional practice.

Professional regulation has something of importance to offer to each of these categories, but only if certain conditions are met. First, the practitioners must understand and accept that, with the privilege of membership there comes the major responsibility of self-regulation. Second, the means of regulation must be appropriate in all respects. It will not be appropriate if the regulatory systems applied are inflexible, concerning themselves with bureaucratic and mechanistic measures while ignoring important matters such as ethical practice, standards and positive outcomes for patients. It will be appropriate, however, if they have at their heart a set of principles which are relevant in a wide variety of circumstances and state a dominant commitment to the public interest.

The International Council of Nurses contribution

In 1985 the International Council of Nurses (ICN) made a major contribution of worldwide application by publishing its document *Report on the Regulation of Nursing: A Report on the Present, A Position for the Future.*[3] This was the culmination of an extensive study undertaken by Margretta Styles to assist ICN to develop a position on the future regulation of nursing. The final chapter of the report sets out the position which ICN then adopted at its Council of National Representatives in 1985. Stated within it is the judgment of the Council that:

> 'The conclusion is inescapable that the welfare of the public, the profession, and the practitioner will be better served if greater relevance, rationality, consistency and clarity are brought to bear upon the regulatory system.'
>
> This is followed by a declaration, the first four clauses of which state that:
>
> 'ICN therefore resolves that a system of governance for the profession must provide for
>
> – high standards for the personal and professional growth and performance of nurses;
> – public sanction for nurses to perform to the extent of their capabilities;
> – participation of the profession in the development of public policy;
> – accountability of the profession to the public for the conduct of its affairs in their behalf.'

This provided the platform from which ICN launched its 'Principles of Professional Regulation' as 'a proposal for a fundamental code regarding regulation of the professions'.

The ICN principles

Twelve years on, in spite of so many changes in and challenges to the arrangements for health care delivery in many parts of the world, these principles remain entirely appropriate. They state that:

(1) regulation should be directed towards an explicit purpose;
(2) regulation should be designed to achieve the stated purpose;
(3) regulatory definitions should be based upon clear definitions of professional scope and accountability;
(4) regulatory definitions and standards should promote the fullest development of the profession commensurate with its potential social contribution;
(5) regulatory systems should recognise and properly incorporate the legitimate roles and interests of interested parties – public, profession and its members, government, employers, other professions – in aspects of standard-setting and administration;
(6) the design of the regulatory system should acknowledge and appropriately balance interdependent interests;
(7) regulatory systems should provide and be limited to those controls and restrictions necessary to achieve their objectives;
(8) standards and processes of regulation should be sufficiently broad and flexible to achieve their objectives and at the same time permit freedom for innovation, growth, and change;
(9) regulatory systems should operate in the most efficient manner, ensuring coherence and coordination among their parts;
(10) regulatory systems should promote universal standards of performance and foster professional identity and mobility to the fullest possible extent compatible with local needs and circumstances;
(11) regulatory processes should provide honest and just treatment for those parties regulated;
(12) in standards and processes regulatory systems should recognise the equality and interdependence of professions.

From these statements of principle a number of important conclusions can naturally flow. The ICN's 1985 statement included some very important and relevant conclusions. By way of illustration, and to reinforce my arguments earlier in this chapter, I quote just a few of them. For example, in respect of 'purpose', that 'The central purpose of statutory regulation of nursing should be to protect the public by ensuring competent, accessible nursing care'; in respect of 'relevance', that 'the regulatory system should include those features necessary to make certain that practitioners maintain knowledge, skills, attitudes and practice in accord with current health needs'; and in respect of 'ultimacy', that 'Since the function of a profession, by definition, is to serve society, nursing and other professions should be encouraged to reach their greatest capacities to serve. As the complexities of health care and its social milieu increase, so must the capabilities of nurses, as citizens and practitioners, be heightened to meet new challenges'.

I am entirely comfortable with these three important statements, as I am with many of the other conclusions in this important ICN publication. Following the publication of this seminal document, the ICN held a series of workshops over a three-year period in several continents to promote understanding of the principles and policy objectives and to equip participants to return to their own countries to either seek improvements in existing arrangements for professional regulation or to press for the introduction of such arrangements where none had previously existed. A study of the quarterly volumes of the World Health Organisation's *International Digest of Health Legislation*[4] for the period 1988 to 1993 inclusive reveals that, in that period alone, legislation to either introduce nursing regulation or improve previous arrangements was passed in 52 countries. I detect a clear cause-and-effect relationship here.

The principles of professional regulation enunciated by ICN in 1985 remain valid 12 years on, as do the main policy objectives that stem from them. It has to be accepted, however, that the context of professional practice has changed substantially in many countries of the world as new systems for organising the delivery of health care have emerged, often increasing substantially the challenges which professional practitioners have to face and resolve. I have therefore been pleased that ICN has recently renewed its consideration of this important subject and produced a new position statement, adhering to the previously stated principles, but supporting them with some revised policy objectives and supportive narrative more appropriate to the final years of the twentieth century. This new text is reproduced as Appendix 7.

While professional regulation composes, as the 1985 ICN publication put it, 'the forms and processes whereby order, consistency and control are brought to an occupation and its practice', it is something greater than that. It is also a substantial part of the means by which an occupation which adopts the worthy title 'profession' demonstrates and honours its accountability to the public and its associated commitment to serve the public interest. For the nursing profession, as for any other profession serving the public interest, an appropriate and effective system of professional regulation should not be seen as a distraction from professional practice, but as an essential element of such practice.

Positive benefits

Provided the regulatory system that a country puts in place for the regulation of nursing is appropriate in all respects, and provided also that it is used as intended by those charged with that responsibility, I claim that it can afford major benefits. I contend that:

(1) it assists governments as they seek to honour their obligations to their citizens;
(2) it provides assurance for employers of nurses that those practitioners have satisfied and continue to satisfy the registration requirements of the regulatory body by which they can be called to account;
(3) it provides for nurses a status that is widely recognised and understood and affords them mobility as practitioners; and
(4) it affords the public, wherever in a country they may reside, with a reasonable assurance of consistently good standards of practice delivered by accountable practitioners.

These I regard as important benefits. They serve to reinforce my conviction that the regulation of nursing is an important matter. I reiterate, however, that they cannot be obtained if the regulatory system is excessively rigid and limiting, and concerns itself with mechanistic measures while ignoring the important criteria of standards, quality, ethical practice and good outcomes. Conversely, they can be achieved if the regulatory

system is founded on a set of sound principles that have as their central theme a dominant commitment to the public interest.

References

1 Pyne R.H. (1994) Unpublished paper
2 *Code of Professional Conduct for the Nurse, Midwife and Health Visitor*. Third Edition (1992). London: UKCC.
3 *Report on the Regulation of Nursing: A Report on the Present, A Position for the Future* (1985). Geneva: International Council of Nurses.
4 *International Digest of Health Legislation (1988 to 1993)*. Geneva: World Health Organisation.

Chapter 3

The Concept of Professional Discipline

Chapter 1 concluded with reference to the profession's responsibility for regulating itself and the importance within that activity of the self-discipline of its members. This chapter seeks to explore the concept of professional discipline that was touched upon in the closing words.

What is professional discipline? Is it concerned with professional ethics or conduct or standards of practice? Possibly these questions, as with those asked at the beginning of Chapter 1, may be best approached by considering first a negative aspect of the subject. I do not mean that we should, at this stage, consider the consequences of a lack of discipline on the part of members of the nursing, midwifery, and health visiting professions: the concerns I have about that lack and the evidence on which those concerns are based will emerge in subsequent chapters. The negative aspect that I have in mind is rather that as we educate aspiring practitioners in the theory and practice of the profession and as we introduce them to the role that they must fulfil as qualified professional practitioners, we so often fail to develop in them an understanding of what professional accountability means.

This conclusion was well illustrated by the case of a psychiatric nurse who appeared before the Professional Conduct Committee of the UKCC to answer charges alleging misconduct resulting from his conviction in a criminal court of cultivating cannabis plants at his home and possessing a quantity of medicines that were the property of his health authority employer. (The medicines were mild analgesics, expectorants and vitamins.) When asked by a member of the Committee that was to decide whether he should retain or lose the right to practise, how he viewed the matter in retrospect he, like so many others, gave an answer which was based only on the effect it had on him and his life. There was no evident appreciation of the significance of his contravention of the law, his casual self-medication or of the damage to the public's trust in the profession that might have resulted from the publicity about his court appearance. He simply said that he was foolish, because he had lost a good job that was convenient to his home and with quite good pay.

Another case which illustrates the same failure to understand what professional accountability means and involves, featured a registered general nurse employed as charge nurse in a large general hospital. He also had appeared in a criminal court and been convicted, on his own plea of guilty, of dishonestly obtaining a quantity of analgesic tablets on two occasions, these being the property of his health authority employer. It emerged that he had a friend who suffered from arthritis, for which this medication had been regularly prescribed. On two occasions that friend, having failed to obtain a further prescription in time, found his supply exhausted and asked the nurse (who became the respondent in the case) to obtain some tablets for him. He readily acquiesced. To obtain a supply he made out a patient's treatment chart for a fictional patient and signed it himself, forging a doctor's signature. The matter came to light when, having obtained a second supply in the same way, he was careless enough to leave the fictitious treatment chart on the office desk where it was found by the doctor whose forged signature it bore.

When you have considered Chapter 8 and Appendix 6 you might care to consider, how, had you been a member of the Professional Conduct Committee, you would have chosen to conclude these two cases.

Would you regard the nurses who were the subject of these cases as guilty of indiscipline, irresponsibility or a failure to honour their accountability? Are these, perhaps, the same thing? There may be some merit in turning again to the same dictionaries (accessed for the purposes of Chapter 1) to assist in arriving at some definition of our terms.

Discipline

First, *discipline*. Unfortunately those dictionaries prove no more helpful with this word than they did with the word *profession*. I say this because, where the word is used as a noun, it tends for the most part to be identified with other words and phrases that do not really approach the interpretation that members of recognised professions would seek. For example, the word is variously identified as 'instruction', 'order', 'mortification', 'punishment', 'training that moulds the mental faculties', 'training in the practice of arms' and others in similar vein. While I accept that all these words and phrases are valid in defining *discipline*, they do not satisfy my requirements as I seek for an explanation of 'professional discipline'.

Buried within the larger definitions, however, there are some points that do help, even if they are not entirely satisfactory. For instance, 'mode of life in accordance with rules', 'orderly or prescribed pattern of behaviour', 'a rule or system of rules governing conduct or activity', 'a system of rules for conduct' and 'self-control'.

In spite of the fact that some of these definitions seem to describe some controlling features of nursing from which it has been necessarily striving to break free, that does, I suggest, take us forward at least a little. If, at this stage, I have to particularise as to why I am not entirely satisfied I would state that it is because of the emphasis on 'rules'. In respect of any occupational or vocational group which can rightly claim the name *profession* I maintain that the rules are concerned with the structure within which the profession is managed and operates and should not be used to define acceptable and unacceptable behaviour. What is acceptable or unacceptable behaviour has to be decided by considering it in its context.

Professional misconduct

With the passing of each year of my direct involvement with the profession's disciplinary machinery I have become more convinced that to respond to the pressures that are often applied to define professional misconduct by producing a list of proscribed actions would be dangerous, since the circumstances in which incidents raise the question 'Is this misconduct in a professional sense?' are rarely the same. For example, although in the vast majority of situations it would be quite wrong to disclose information received from a patient in confidence, there are rare and exceptional circumstances in which it would be right to do so. Therefore to ensure in statutory rules a list of actions and omissions that are considered misconduct, and should therefore lead to removal from the register, would be bad both for members of the profession and members of the public.

It would be unsatisfactory and unjust for members of the profession if the context of an alleged offence (often unreasonable by virtue of excessive pressure of work, unclear policies, inadequate management, etc.) were not to be considered before labelling an episode of behaviour 'professional misconduct'. For the public who depend upon the availability of a competent and caring service from persons on the UKCC's register, it would also be unsatisfactory because no list prepared now could possibly cater for all the eventualities in as little as 5 years' time. Could our predecessors have possibly contemplated the need to include in such a list attempts to unreasonably resist patients' access to their records, for example? I doubt it very much. The inevitable conclusion drawn by those faced with the task of producing such a list would be that it had to be produced in such general terms that it would be better to have no such document at all. Besides, would such a closely defined set of rules on 'misconduct' (even if it could be kept up to date, which is unlikely in the extreme) be consistent with membership of a profession whose practitioners must be constantly engaged in the exercise of personal judgment, and in an often imperfect environment? I contend that it would not.

Responsibility

Now to the word *responsibility*. Here I find my dictionaries more to my liking, since they clearly indicate (a) that to be responsible is to be obliged, either legally or morally, to take care of something or to carry out a duty, and (b) that one is liable to be blamed for failure. Surely these are things about which nurses, midwives and health visitors know a great deal and which they accept as a necessary consequence of their professional status.

Lack of responsibility, however, is not something that is manifested only by practitioners in direct clinical practice. Those who have accepted the different responsibility associated with nursing, midwifery or health visiting managerial positions often reveal it just as strongly. When that happens the consequences may be still more serious, because the manager who fails to act responsibly not only adversely affects the service to patients or clients but creates a situation in which his or her own staff may be put at risk. The consequences may be made heavier still if a decision is made which seeks a short-term solution to the problem with no thought for the long-term consequences.

One case heard by the Professional Conduct Committee in the United Kingdom which illustrates this phenomenon involved a 33-year-old registered general nurse who had been employed as the senior sister in an intensive therapy unit. She had been found staggering about in the unit early one afternoon and, when asked what was wrong by a colleague, said that she had ingested two or three sodium amytal tablets from a bottle which had been in the possession of a patient admitted earlier that day. On the face of it this appeared to be a serious offence on the part of the sister. The evidence of the background to the incident, however, revealed her as more victim than villain.

It emerged that, some months earlier, the nurse manager to whom this sister had line responsibility had to be admitted to hospital for a planned major operation. It was known that she would be absent for several months. It was also known that no cover for her duties could be organised. The more senior nurse manager admitted that they took stock of their position. They agreed that this sister was totally reliable and that they need not worry themselves about that unit, instead concentrating their stretched management resources in those areas where the sisters were, in their view, less reliable or experienced.

The sister's normal link to more senior management had gone. In no time at all the pressure on her increased as the unit became progressively more busy; there was severe staff shortage, little continuity, and the staff she had were often of inadequate quality or experience. Being the kind of person she was – highly skilled and committed – the sister waited for her managers to notice her dilemma rather than telling them. So she began and continued to work quite excessive hours to keep the unit going and stopped leaving the unit for meal breaks. Nobody seemed to notice the stress to which she was subject or how terribly tired she was.

On the day of the incident, once again she did not leave the unit for lunch, but simply snatched a few minutes for a cup of coffee in the staff room. It was then that she swallowed the tablets which (inevitably in her tired condition) acted very quickly. She tried to return to her duties but her condition led a colleague to call a senior nurse manager. Then that manager became aware of just how great were the burdens this sister had been bearing – so great that when they removed her they had to close the unit.

Once the full picture had been seen and understood the immediate managers were kind and helpful. They channelled the sister to appropriate medical help and reassured her about her future employment. They also involved the support of the Nurses Welfare Service about which you can read in Chapter 10. Her appearance before the Professional Conduct Committee resulted from a complaint by a more senior manager.

That case illustrates the type of problem that can develop for a practitioner who is too compliant, too submissive and lacking in assertiveness. It also illustrates that management is not simply about waiting to be told about the problems but walking the job so that they are identified. It can be recorded that the immediate managers in this case recognised their failure and learnt from the experience. It is not always so, as the following example illustrates.

A 28-year-old registered general nurse became the subject of a Professional Conduct Committee hearing following a conviction in a magistrates court for theft of a considerable quantity of pethidine, fortral, syringes and needles from the company for which she worked as an occupational health nurse. A psychiatrist's report, submitted to the committee in evidence, revealed that a year earlier, when employed as a ward sister, she had been discovered misappropriating tranquillising drugs from her ward stock. She had (the report indicated) been quietly asked to resign, in return for which the nurse managers would take no further action on the matter. She did resign and quickly found employment with the heavy engineering company where controlled drugs were (of necessity) stocked and the control system (regrettably) was almost non-existent. The consequences you have been told.

This was a case in which the nurse concerned was not the only one who failed to act responsibly. Those nurse managers also have much to answer for since, in seeking a short-term solution to their immediate problem and thus succeeding in their desire to avoid any bad publicity for 'their hospital', they abrogated most aspects of their professional responsibility. In disposing of this nurse from their employment but doing nothing further either to channel her to help or to question her continued appropriateness to be a registered nurse they were simply (to put the best possible interpretation on it) acting to protect their particular patients at that time. Meanwhile, however, they were neglecting their responsibilities to their profession and its standards and they were neglecting their responsibilities for this possibly sick colleague. By their failure the public were put at risk and this colleague was allowed to progress further into drug dependence, then requiring more time and much more medical and social work help to achieve her rehabilitation.

After reading Chapter 7 you might care to analyse the behaviour of all the participants in the cases described above. One of the lessons to emerge is certainly that while professional nurses, midwives and health visitors are accountable for their own actions, and while those practitioners who take up managerial posts bear special responsibilities which relate both to the public and to members of the profession, all members of the profession have responsibility to care for and about each other.

Unfortunately, although there is evidence that it has been changing for the better in recent years, it seems that there are still too many practitioners who choose to look the other way or not to interfere when they suspect or know that a colleague is behaving unprofessionally. Quite apart from the fact that this allows that colleague to go on putting herself at risk, it places patients at risk from a possibly unsafe practitioner. Some registered practitioners, by their unquestioning response to certain requests and by their willingness to disregard carefully prepared policies, so often unwittingly fail their colleagues, their profession and (most of all) their patients and clients. Just one more illustration must suffice.

A staff nurse on night duty in a large city general hospital expressed concern that another nurse was 'borrowing' pethidine from her ward very often, and suggested to the night manager that the ward in question ought to organise itself better so that the night staff did not need to 'borrow' a drug that was in frequent use. This innocent report led to an investigation which revealed that another registered nurse had been obtaining pethidine not only from that ward but also from many other wards in this large hospital. Still more, it revealed that the 'borrowing' was taking place when the ward's stock was more than adequate to respond to the current prescriptions. This very large amount of pethidine (on average 700 mg each night shift worked over several months) was illegally and fraudulently obtained by the nurse by the simple expedient of going to other wards with treatment cards of fictitious patients and stating 'I have to give this patient some pethidine and I have run out. Can I borrow some?' In ward after ward, other registered nurses were providing the pethidine, recording its administration in their ward drug recording book and signing as having witnessed the administration when all they had witnessed was another nurse leaving the ward with an ampoule and a treatment card for a non-existent patient. And all this in a hospital which had a good, specific and easily available policy concerning the administration of medicines. So much for personal responsibility for one's actions.

Conclusion

So what is professional discipline? Surely it is two things. At the individual level I believe it to be the self-dicipline of the members of the profession – their individual determination to act in a responsible way and in accordance with the moral principles of their profession. At the collective level I see it as the process by which the professions of nursing, midwifery and health visiting (acting not in their own interest but on behalf of the public) operate that section of the law that permits the application of appropriate sanctions to its culpable members impaired by illness.

Sir David Napley, in an address to the veterinary profession in 1987, said:

> 'The characteristic most resented by those who attack the professions – our independence – is the very characteristic of a true profession and that which provides the greatest measure of protection for the public. Independence means an exemption from external control or support.'[1]

To that Joy Wingfield has added:

> 'Independence also implies a voluntary submission by the professional to control and review of his behaviour by his peers.
>
> Although this control must be exercised in a fair and judicial manner, self-discipline is infinitely more demanding than the basic levels of morality established at law.'[2]

Professional discipline is inextricably entwined with the whole theme of responsibility. This is one of eight key words around which Baroness Macfarlane built an article in 1980 as she expressed her hopes for nursing in the decade then to come. That decade has now passed, but the words remain valid and applicable in any decade. In that article it was stated that:

> 'We also have a responsibility for our own professional actions. This is legally a fact, but as professionals we make decisions about the nursing care of individuals and we must be seen to be accountable for the clinical decisions we make and the actions we carry out. A developing sense of professional responsibility and accountability for clinical nursing actions by the practising nurse are priorities as we enter the next decade.'[3]

I was delighted when that article was first published to read such a positive statement, since we so often think and speak in negative terms when the subject is 'discipline' or 'responsibility'. To be self-disciplined and to act responsibly are positive virtues, since without them all the knowledge and skill we possess will consistently fail to provide care of a high standard.

Looking back, I also find it significant that Baroness Macfarlane wrote of 'being seen to be accountable' and of 'accountability for clinical nursing actions'. Those words 'accountable' and 'accountability' have been the subject of a great deal of exploration and elaboration in recent years. The basis of that interest is a feature of Chapter 7.

References

1 Sir David Napley. *Veterinary Record*, 1987; **121**, 281.
2 Joy Wingfield. Misconduct and the pharmacist. *The Pharmaceutical Journal*, 27 October 1990.
3 Baroness Macfarlane. *Nursing Mirror*, 10 January 1980.

Section II

The Law Relating to Professional Regulation

Chapter 4

Registration and Regulation – Its Origins and Development

Statutory control of nursing, midwifery and health visiting education and practice has not always existed in the form we know it today. The Nurses, Midwives and Health Visitors Act, which Parliament approved and which received the Royal Assent in 1979, became fully operative on 1 July 1983. On that date an entirely new structure came into existence and operation, with new bodies completely replacing old. Significantly, however, the new registration and regulatory body is possessed of important new powers which are the subject of Chapters 5, 6 and 9. This 1979 Act was again substantially amended by the Nurses, Midwives and Health Visitors Act of 1992, which became operative in part later in the same year, and in full in 1993. This new legislation remedied a number of deficits in the 1979 Act which had been experienced in its operation.

Origins

Before proceeding to consideration of the new legislation there is merit in taking a brief look back. This is not suggested as an exercise in nostalgia, but as one way of remembering just how precious our professional inheritance in the United Kingdom is and how great is our responsibility to the future. It is now well over 100 years since the fight for the registration of nurses and midwives seriously began, yet it is easy to observe the various ways in which the concept of 'profession' is still under attack: time indeed to consider the past in order to value the present and prepare for the future.

In 1874, Miss Florence Lees published her book entitled *A Handbook for Ward Sisters*. For the purpose of this chapter, that book is significant because of three short sentences in the preface by Dr (later Sir) Henry Acland, rather than for its main contents. Dr Acland wrote:

> 'The Medical Act of 1858 allows women to be registered as medical practitioners. It makes no provision for the registration of trained nurses. That this ought to be remedied can hardly admit of doubt.'

Even though he was President of the General Medical Council when the book was published, his view that 'it can hardly admit of doubt' was not shared by all within his own profession or, indeed, by all nurses. Many immediately expressed their reservations. Doubts surfaced in plenty and, over the years that followed – particularly during the period 1880 to 1900, the opposing factions furiously debated their various views. The events of this period as they apply to both nursing and midwifery are dealt with at length in two chapters in *Nursing and Midwifery since 1900* (edited by Allan and Jolley).[1] For the present purposes of this chapter it must suffice to state that the first 'Midwives Act' reached the statute book in 1902 and (after some delay because the House of Commons took excessive time on the Dogs Protection Bill) the Nurses Registration Acts, applying the registration and regulation principles to the countries of the United Kingdom, followed in 1919. Formal registration of Health Visitors came only with the Nurses, Midwives and Health Visitors Act 1979, operative from 1983.

The fascinating details of those years and of the traumatic early life of the General Nursing Council for England and Wales are described in the books listed at the end of this chapter, to which the enthusiastic student of legislation or nursing and midwifery history can refer.[2,3,4] It is a matter of record, however, that one of the responsibilities placed upon the now replaced statutory bodies by those 1902 and 1919 Acts of Parliament, and which continues to be placed with the United Kingdom Central Council for Nursing, Midwifery and Health Visiting by the Nursing, Midwives and Health Visitors Act of 1979, is that aspect of professional regulation known as professional discipline: the means by which a person can, in the public interest, be removed from the register and thus prevented from practising as a nurse, midwife or health visitor.

It can be seen, therefore, that from the time when the law first introduced a new regime for training, examination and approval of training institutions, it also required the same bodies it established to undertake not only that work in the public interest but also to exercise a professional disciplinary function. Peer judgment had arrived as an aspect of the law. If a nurse was a subject of complaint which called into question her nurse registration status, it would be primarily nurses who would hear the evidence and decide whether her right to practise should be removed. From the outset the statutory bodies (i.e. the General Nursing Councils and Central Midwives Boards) exercised this important function for the protection of the public, not for the self-aggrandisement of their respective professions.

The new legislation of 1979 replaced five bodies which had exercised the disciplinary function for one professional group, one country or both profession and country. In my brief retrospective study I use, for illustrative purposes, the former General Nursing Council for England and Wales.

At first, and indeed for many years, all cases were first considered by the Disciplinary and Penal Cases Committee, the members of which had to decide whether a *prima facie* case of misconduct had been established. Where the decision was in the affirmative the case was then considered at a full Council meeting to determine whether or not to remove the practitioner from the register. The disadvantage of this system is clear in retrospect. When a case was forwarded for a hearing, those members already aware of the circumstances because of their membership of the Disciplinary and Penal Cases Committee would now participate in judgment of the same case – a procedure seen to be unsatisfactory over the years. Eventually (though not until the Nurses Act of 1969) the law ensured that, if a case were to go right through the professional disciplinary system, it would be subjected to the consideration of two entirely separate groups of members.

The records of the Disciplinary and Penal Cases Committee over the early years of the life of the former General Nursing Council for England and Wales make fascinating reading, as do the Council minutes which record the charges against those referred for possible removal of their names from the register and the decisions that resulted from those hearings. They present a fragment of rather specialised social history, and reveal something of the attitudes of the members of this new registered profession to their allegedly delinquent peers.

As in the previous editions of this book, I draw attention to the first 30 cases considered by the Committee, most of which were referred on to the Council for hearing. You must derive your own conclusions as to whether the judgments made were harsh or lenient, whether they were those required for public protection or rather to pronounce a moral judgment or to punish the nurse.

Theft from shops

We tend to assume that 'shoplifting' is a phenomenon of post-Second World War society and the emergence of tempting displays in large department stores and supermarkets. It might seem surprising, therefore, that 12 of the first 30 cases (in the 1920s) involved theft from shops. Five resulted from the theft of hats from the same large London store. The remainder involved yet more ladies' hats and other items of clothing.

Eleven of the 12 respondent nurses were removed from the register. The remaining one – a deputy matron – received powerful mitigating support from the matron, the chairman of the hospital board (a magistrate) and senior medical staff. Such evidence of rallying to the aid of a convicted nurse rather than dismissing her instantly was rare in those early days of nurse registration.

Cases concerning personal conduct

Seven of the first 30 cases mentioned above were concerned with the personal conduct, completely separate from their places of employment, of the persons about whom the complaints were made. Four of the seven were removed from the register. Their 'offences' were, respectively, 'bearing two illegitimate children', 'living in adultery', 'misconduct with a man in an hotel', and 'drunk and disorderly in a public place'. Two of the remaining three were formally warned about their behaviour. One had been reported for 'betting in a public house' and the other for 'making an unauthorised collection for a good cause'. The remaining nurse had no action taken against him following a report that he had left his wife. The reader might care to compare the cases in this list with the information provided in Appendix 6.

Cases concerning patients or their property

Three cases only fell into this category. All culminated in removal from the register. One involved the theft of a diamond ring and £5 (a large sum of money in 1925) from a patient. The others involved theft of money from the property of deceased patients.

Cases concerned with employment

One nurse was removed from the register for forging a character reference to support her application for a nursing post. The other two respondent nurses in this category were also removed from the register, one for being drunk on duty and the other for being found asleep on night duty.

Cases involving theft from employers or colleagues

Three further nurses found their names removed from the register for offences of this kind. One concerned theft from her employer (of food that she argued would otherwise have gone to waste). The other two were the result of theft from colleagues – a dress and a watch respectively.

Other cases

The remaining two nurses to feature in the first 30 cases to be considered by the former General Nursing Council for England and Wales were also the subject of 'removal from the register' decisions. The first was the result of the theft of £11 from some family friends. The second, and the last of the 30 cases to which I am referring in this short retrospective study, was the first to involve drugs in any way. The particular offence is described in the Council's records as 'taking and unlawfully possessing morphine'.

A number of conclusions can be drawn from reference to the first 30 cases. Two that leap from the page are that the removal rate was high (86%) and that many of those removed were so 'removed' for reasons which had little or nothing to do with their professional work.

On the latter point, I noted with great interest that, as early as case 3 (the first reported hat theft) the Council was subjected to pressure from one of the major nursing membership organisations of the day. Its secretary wrote that the Council *must* remove this lady from the register 'to maintain the purity of the profession'. She was removed, and the phrase 'to maintain the purity of the profession' slipped into the Council's language when notifying removal and remained there for many years to come.

I found it surprising, as I researched this subject, that certain of the types of case that were culminating in removal from the register in the period up to 1930 were still being similarly resolved in the 1940s. For example, one nurse was removed from the register in 1943 in that 'being unmarried, she gave birth to a child'.

The fact is, however, that a regulatory system had been established and brought into operation. It might be felt that I am implying criticism of those charged in the early years of nurse registration with determining whether a person should lose or retain the right to practise. My response to that would be to say that I imagine that those involved as Council members probably had opinions that were not unlike those of society at large. It seems clear that the context in which an incident occurred was not generally taken into account in those early years. This steadily changed during ensuing years, thus enabling the Council's members and senior professional officers to exert considerable influence on the form of the relevant clauses of the Bill that became the

Nurses, Midwives and Health Visitors Act 1979, and still more in the development of the 1992 Act which amended it.

The exertion of such influence extended not only to seeking legislation that improved the means by which the profession could regulate itself in the public interest. It was also aimed at replacing the silence and ambiguity of the old legislation with a mandatory requirement to establish and improve standards of professional conduct and the power to give advice to that end. That pressure succeeded. The importance and impact of the change has given to the system and procedures of professional regulation a new and positive emphasis.

References

1 *Nursing and Midwifery since 1900*. Edited by Allan and Jolley. London: Faber and Faber. Particularly Chapter 2 by R.H. Pyne; Chapter 14 by E.A. Bent.

2 Bendall E.R.D & Raybould E. (1969) *History of the General Nursing Council for England and Wales, 1919–1969*. London: H.K. Lewis and Co.

3 Abel-Smith B. (1960) *A History of the Nursing Profession*. London: Heineman Educational Books Ltd.

4 *The Work of Mrs Bedford Fenwick and the Rise of Professional Nursing* (1973). London: The Royal College of Nursing.

Chapter 5

The Legal Basis of the Regulation of the Nursing, Midwifery and Health Visiting Professions

In July 1983, the means by which the nursing, midwifery and health visiting professions in the United Kingdom were regulated underwent its most significant change for many years when the Nurses, Midwives and Health Visitors Act which Parliament had passed into law in 1979[1] at last became fully operative. The system which this Act created was described in the previous edition of this book. At the time that this legislation became fully operative a commitment to review its operation and effectiveness after 5 years was made by the relevant Government department – the Department of Health. That commitment was honoured and, as a result of the review, further legislation eventually came before Parliament in 1991, and, after certain amendments in the course of its progress through the Parliamentary system, became law in 1992.[2] This revised law, designed to eliminate what had been seen as a number of defects in the 1979 legislation, became fully operative in 1993. It amends the 1979 Act, but leaves many of its clauses intact. Until Parliamentary time is found to consider and approve a consolidated version of the two Acts, it is necessary to consider the composite effect of both.

In the manner of its construction, the United Kingdom's legislation encompasses the essential elements of a professional regulatory system described in Chapter 1 and is built around most of the principles for regulation described in Chapter 2.

The Nurses, Midwives and Health Visitors Acts 1979 and 1992

The functions of the body established by this law to regulate the professions in the United Kingdom (the full title of which is the United Kingdom Central Council for Nurses, Midwives and Health Visitors) are set out in section 2 of the 1979 Act. This section, amended only modestly by the 1992 Act, now states that:

'(1) The principal functions of the Central Council shall be to establish and improve standards of training and professional conduct for nurses, midwives and health visitors.

(2) The Council shall ensure that the standards of training they establish are such as to meet any Community (meaning the European Union) standards of the United Kingdom.

(3) The Council shall by means of rules determine the conditions of a person's

being admitted to training, and the kind, content and standard of training to be undertaken, with a view to registration.

(4) The rules may also make provision with respect to the kind and standard of further training available for those persons who are already registered.

(5) The powers of the Council shall include that of providing, in such manner as it thinks fit, advice for nurses, midwives and health visitors on standards of professional conduct.

(6) In the discharge of its functions the Council shall have a proper regard for the interests of all groups within the professions, including those with minority representation.'[3]

Further functions concerning important aspects of professional regulation are to be found in subsequent sections of the same Act, but modified and enhanced in some instances by clauses in the 1992 Act which introduce significant modifications and some important new powers. These other functions are concerned with such important matters as the means by which a person can achieve registration as a nurse, midwife or health visitor, the maintenance and use of the professional register and removal or suspension from the register, all of this satisfying the essential elements referred to in Chapter 2.

It can be readily seen from this list of functions set out in section 2 of the 1979 Act, and the major functions covered by other sections of both Acts, that this legislation is concerned with public protection and the wider public interest. It is not intended to protect the professions, or to enhance their status, though both of these might be beneficial by-products of its correct and committed operation by the Council members and its staff.

The 1979 Act required the establishment, in each of the four countries of the United Kingdom, of a National Board for Nursing, Midwifery and Health Visiting. The functions of the Boards were revised to some degree by the 1992 Act, and now read in legislation as follows:

'(1) The National Boards shall in England, Wales, Scotland and Northern Ireland respectively –

(a) approve institutions in relation to provision of –

(i) courses of training with a view to enabling persons to qualify for registration as nurses, midwives or health visitors or for the recording of additional qualifications in the register; and

(ii) courses of further training for those already registered;

(b) ensure that such courses meet the requirements of the Central Council as to their kind, content and standard;

(c) hold or arrange for others to hold, such examinations as are necessary to enable persons to satisfy requirements for registration or to obtain additional qualifications;

(d) collaborate with the Council in the promotion of improved training methods; and

(e) perform such other functions relating to nurses, midwives or health visitors as the Secretary of State may by order prescribe.

(2) The National Boards shall discharge their functions subject to and in

accordance with any applicable rules of the Council and shall take account of any difference in the considerations applying to the different professions.'[4]

The major change to this list of functions effected by the 1992 Act was that the function of investigating allegations of misconduct and deciding whether or not they needed referral to the Council was removed from the Boards, thus placing the entire professional disciplinary process with the Council which, in any case, had always been required to meet the total cost of this activity from registration and other fee income. The first of the functions listed above was also changed to reflect modifications in the arrangements for the provision of education for the professions. Previously the Boards had been required to 'provide, or arrange for others to provide' courses. Another change in the list of functions, and one of potential significance, was the introduction of clause (1)(e). The Board cannot take unto itself new functions, but will be required to if the relevant Government Minister so prescribes in a Ministerial Order.

It can be seen from these passages of legislation that the Boards must operate within the constraints that both the primary law and the Council through rules (i.e. the secondary or subordinate law which it prepares and which receives approval through a simple Parliamentary process) prescribe. The National Boards therefore bear an accountability both to their linked Government Departments from which they receive much of their funding and to the Council whose requirements in specific respects, set out in law, they must satisfy.

Membership of the Council and Boards

The 1992 Act introduced major changes in both the Council and Boards membership structure and the means by which people make their way into membership. Prior to this change, the Boards had membership varying from 35 (Northern Ireland) to 45 (England). Two-thirds of that number was composed of persons elected by the professions' members in the respective country, the remainder being appointed by Government Ministers. As a result of the 1992 Act the Board membership is much smaller and the Chairman and all other non-executive members of it are appointed by Government Ministers. The result is a Board membership composed of both non-executive and executive members, in many respects like the Trust Boards responsible for much of the National Health Service as it is now constructed in the United Kingdom. Certain specific requirements of the law have to be satisfied in the making of appointments to a Board, not least that a majority of the members must be registered nurses, midwives or health visitors.

The same legislation which removed the elected component from the membership of the Boards introduced it into the membership of the Council. Previously a Board, as then constructed, nominated seven of its members to serve on the Council, while retaining their Board membership. To the 28 members from this source were added a further 17 members appointed by the Secretary of State, creating a Council membership of 45. As a result of the 1992 Act, the Council now (since April 1993) has a membership, two-thirds of which is elected by members of the professions with current and effective registration, the remaining one-third being appointed by the Secretary of State for Health, after wide consultation. The same legislation allows that the number of members may be up to a maximum of 60, but a number divisible by 3 to allow the two-thirds/one-third criterion to be met, and permits the Council to determine the number. To the present time it has chosen the maximum membership figure, requiring the election of 40 members who are practising nurses, midwives or health visitors and the appointment by Government Ministers (after wide consultation) of 20 members.

It has to be assumed that the original membership arrangements were sought by the Government of the day and approved by Parliament in the belief that they would create a corporate structure in which the determination of educational policy and its effective implementation was rendered relatively simple, since 28 of the members responsible for determining policy were also members of the Boards which were responsible for its implementation. It did not, however, operate well in practice. One difficulty was that the Boards provided a majority of the members of the Council to which they were accountable for significant aspects of their work, so were in effect in a position to monitor themselves. Another was that, while the 28 Board members who were also Council members could, if they worked together, command a majority in a Council vote, they constituted only a small minority when they returned to their respective Boards. When the Board members were not operating in harmony, the debates in Council tended to become both long and stagnant, creating a great feeling of frustration. Many of those who bore the burden of dual membership found that it created for them both difficulty and tension. Meanwhile, those who were directly appointed as Council members found the whole experience frustrating in the extreme, since it was often extremely difficult if not impossible to move forward the business of the Council in respect of professional education and training at anything like an acceptable pace.

For those in dual membership there was yet another essentially practical problem. It was that of trying to find sufficient time to contribute fully to the work of both the Council and their particular Board while, at the same time, holding full-time salaried posts. This was a totally unreasonable burden. Not surprisingly, the list of absentees from meetings at which key policy debates were taking place was often substantial. It was an arrangement that, though only introduced in 1983, was seen by 1992 to have more negative than positive effects and to be overdue for replacement.

Under the new arrangements introduced by the 1992 Act there is no dual membership and therefore no members of either Council or Boards who are subjected to the stress or the excessive demands on their time that the former arrangements created. That is not to say that either Board or Council membership is a sinecure. It demands commitment in every respect, and consumes a great deal of an individual's personal time, even if fortunate enough to be allowed substantial time off for Board or Council business by an employer who appreciates the importance of professional regulation. To say that things are better should not be interpreted as stating that the membership structure of the Council is perfect. The reader will find further comment on this subject in a later chapter.

Roles and responsibilities

The functions of the National Boards under the legislation as now composed are exactly those set out in the relevant section of the 1979 Act, as amended by the 1992 Act, which has been set out above. They are about control of the route to the professional register and the standards to be attained in order to achieve registration. They are about applying the same controls and standards to the acquisition of further professional qualifications that can be recorded as supplements to a person's registration entry. They are about assisting to achieve the improvements in training methods and outcomes that the Council wishes to see achieved. They involve an accountability to the Council which was both less apparent and less easy to achieve under the previous arrangements.

The responsibilities are clearly constrained, yet provide for the Boards an extremely important function to perform and contribution to make to the regulation of the profession, since control of admission to the professional register is one of the essential elements of professional regulation without which that register loses its significance.

While the United Kingdom legislation, as now composed, limits the Boards to a small number of important functions, it allows for the Council a much less constrained role. It is specific in its requirements that the Council create and maintain a professional register, control admission to the register (both through the requirements it imposes on Boards in respect of those undertaking education and training in the UK and its own procedures to evaluate applicants whose original registration is in a country outside the UK) and have in place arrangements whereby registration can be removed or suspended, all of which are public interest functions. But it also leaves enormous scope for freedom and initiative in stating, at section 2(1) of the 1979 Act, that:

> 'The principal functions of the Central Council shall be to establish and improve standards of training and professional conduct for nurses, midwives and health visitors.'

There can be very few sentences in British law to compare with this. In a sentence of only 25 words, set out on the face of an Act of Parliament, the legislators have used those important words *principal*, *shall* and *improve*. Note, not just to 'establish', but 'improve', which I take to mean continually or perpetually improve. Note not 'may', but 'shall'. The improvement referred to is mandatory, not permissive. Note that our legislators in the British Parliament have done the professions a service by placing training and conduct together in a phrase, thus providing a reminder that the standards of the latter are, to a significant degree, a product of the standards of the former.

There can be no doubt that this is not legislation that is about going backwards or simply standing still. It is most certainly about going forward. The profession in the United Kingdom is fortunate indeed to have such a clause in the legislation concerning regulation of the profession, and must not allow it to become redundant for lack of use. It sets a new, challenging, forward-looking, standards-related tone and the requirement that the specific functions prescribed later in the Act be performed against this positive background.

In respect of education and training, the Council has responded to this challenge. It has done so through the introduction of a new means of preparation for registration and practice. To that it has more recently added the requirement that, in order to maintain the right to practise through renewal of registration each third year, an individual must produce evidence of the study and action undertaken during the preceding registration period to maintain and improve knowledge and skill relative to her or his sphere of practice.

The Council has also made use of its power under this clause concerning 'professional conduct' and the reinforcement it receives from clause 5 of the same section of the Act which states that:

> 'The powers of the Council shall include that of providing, in such manner as it thinks fit, advice for nurses, midwives and health visitors on standards of professional conduct.'

It is not the purpose of this book to elaborate upon either the law concerning preparation for practice and maintaining competence for practice or its implementation, since this has been comprehensively described and explored by other authors. One of its principal purposes is, however, to explore the law, and the operation of the law, whereby, in the public interest, practitioners can be removed or suspended from the register. Another is to explore (principally in Chapters 8 and 9) the steps taken to challenge the professions regulated by the Council in respect of professional conduct and to consider further measures that might usefully be taken to seek to generate an improved understanding of accountability in relation to professional practice. In these respects it aims to make a substantial contribution to the literature concerning professional regulation.

Suffice it for the present to say that, 18 years after it was first passed into law, and 5 years since it was amended by a further Act of Parliament, the professions have yet to grasp fully the significance of the positive legislation it has and to respond comprehensively to the challenges and opportunities it offers.

References

1 *Nurses, Midwives and Health Visitors Act 1979*. London: HMSO.
2 *Nurses, Midwives and Health Visitors Act 1992*. London: HMSO.
3 Section 2 of the *Nurses, Midwives and Health Visitors Act 1979*, as amended by the *Nurses, Midwives and Health Visitors Act 1992*. London: HMSO.
4 Section 6 of the *Nurses, Midwives and Health Visitors Act 1979*, as amended by the *Nurses, Midwives and Health Visitors Act 1992*. London: HMSO.

Chapter 6

The Current Law and its Operation

Introduction

When I prepared the second (1992) edition of this book I used the short chapter which this now replaces to identify and comment upon what I regarded as the significant defects of the law concerning the regulation of the nursing, midwifery and health visiting professions in the United Kingdom as it then stood. I then proceeded to press the case for a number of legislative amendments that I believed would go far towards remedying those identified defects. As I complete this third edition I am pleased to record that, to a substantial degree, those defects have been remedied by the amendments made to the Nurses, Midwives and Health Visitors Act 1979[1] by the 1992 Act of the same name.[2]

Structural problems

I commented upon the structural problems that resulted from the large overlap in membership between the Central Council (UKCC) and the National Boards which imposed impossible burdens on the 28 persons who were in membership of both, while also holding full-time professional posts. That problem was eliminated by legislative amendments that introduced a revised constitution for each of these bodies and rejected the membership overlap arrangements that had been a core feature of the replaced legislation. This has, I believe, had the effect of reducing the burden on individual members while enabling them to address the responsibilities of their respective bodies more satisfactorily.

Responsibility for investigating allegations of misconduct

Coincident with the substantial reduction in the size of National Boards membership there came a significant change in the role of those bodies and the part they played in the regulatory process. This was brought about by the transfer, to the Council, of the responsibility for the investigation of allegations of misconduct. This was another change I had argued was essential if some consistency was to be brought into the process and the cost of it brought under control. I have no doubt that this transfer of responsibility has proved beneficial and has achieved both of the objectives identified.

Professional Conduct Committee delays

Another matter of great concern to me in 1991 was the very serious delay that was evident between the initial report of a criminal conviction or allegation of misconduct and, should it proceed to that stage, the eventual Professional Conduct Committee hearing that might lead to removal of the person's name from the professional register. The public interest was evidently not being served adequately if there was a delay of many months, during all of which time that practitioner could engage in the practice of their profession without any reservation or limitation.

I am pleased to note that the period between initial report and eventual hearing is now much shorter, this being in large part a product of the enormous contribution of the UKCC members who serve at either the sieving stage (the Preliminary Proceedings Committee) or as members of Professional Conduct Committees, and also of the Council's staff and contracted lawyers involved in the preparation of cases. Another major factor in achieving this improvement has been a significant reduction in the number of inappropriate referrals that I identified as a cause of concern in 1991. This has been brought about as a result of two legislative changes. First, the fact that, at the preliminary stage, all cases are considered by one committee of the Council, rather than some being heard by each of the Investigating Committees of the four National Boards, has introduced much greater consistency of decisions. Second, and possibly making an even greater contribution to the improvement, has been the introduction of a power, for the Preliminary Proceedings Committee, where it deems it appropriate to use it, to administer a formal caution rather than refer a person for hearing before the Professional Conduct Committee.

Interim suspension from practice

There are, however, limits to the speed with which cases can be progressed from initial report or complaint through to hearing. Where the cases are not consequent upon a criminal conviction, it is necessary to identify witnesses to the alleged events, meet and take statements from them and build the results into a credible prosecution if, indeed, there is material evidence to make that possible. That evidence has to be made available to the person who is the subject of complaint so that there is no doubt in their mind of the details of the allegation against them and which is calling into question their future registration status. Time has to be allowed for the preparation of a defence. The law requires significant periods of notice of a hearing. Weeks easily become months before a case is ready for hearing.

In the second edition I expressed concern at the absence of any power for the regulatory body, in exceptional cases, where there was deemed to be an immediate risk to the public, to order an interim suspension of registration. I am pleased to record that Parliament acceded to the request to amend the legislation and grant this power. There is good evidence that, since becoming available to the Preliminary Proceedings Committee in 1993, this power has been used responsibly, this to the public benefit. It is, of course, incumbent on the Council, once interim suspension of registration has been imposed, to complete its investigations and bring the case for definitive hearing before the Professional Conduct Committee as quickly as possible. This responsibility has been well recognised, and an arrangement operated whereby any interim suspension is reviewed at frequent intervals while extant.

Suspension from the register

Another of my pleas was for the introduction of a power of suspension from the register (as distinct from removal from the register) for use by the Health Committee. The effect in both cases would be that the person is prevented from practising in their profession, so the objective of public protection would be achieved. My concern was to avoid the stigma of 'removal', which I believe to be appropriate where the reason is proven misconduct, but not appropriate for the person who is to be prevented from practising because her or his fitness to practise has been found to be seriously impaired by illness. Use of the word 'suspension' seemed to avoid, or at least reduce, the risk of such stigmatisation. I am pleased that the small yet significant adjustment to the law to make this possible was carried.

The constitution of Professional Conduct Committees

Another matter of concern to me in 1991 resulted from the wording of section 12(3) of the Nurses, Midwives and Health Visitors Act 1979.[1]

While requiring that a person be judged 'by a committee selected with due regard to the professional field in which that person works or has worked' it also limited membership of the Professional Conduct Committee to members of the Council, therefore sometimes rendering this impossible. Another effect was to limit the size of the pool from which a committee to hear any specific case or set of cases could be convened. I desired to see this changed in order to involve both lay members nominated by recognised consumer organisations and further members of the professions regulated by the Council in this work.

Once again, the legislators in Parliament have addressed this issue, so that the clause, as now amended, states that:

> 'The committees need not be constituted exclusively from members of the Council, but the rules shall provide, in relation to committees constituted by them, that there shall only be a quorum if a majority of those present are members of the Council.'[2]

The 'due regard' criterion continued to apply, but would, it appeared, be easier to honour.

This new clause provided an opportunity to reduce the burdens on members while continuing to have as many meetings of the Professional Conduct Committee as were necessary. It also carried with it the merit of opening this important aspect of professional regulation to greater public participation, this in turn generating increased public confidence in the Council and its procedures. This should, to some degree, reduce the significance of the criticisms expressed by Robinson.[3]

The third potential benefit was that, by involving, in this important regulatory aspect, some members of the professions who were not Council members, a greater understanding of regulation would permeate through their ranks and the salutary lessons to be derived from the hearings would be made more widely available.

To my considerable surprise, the Council seemed surprisingly coy about passing through the door that the law had opened for it. It was slow to take the first step of increased lay participation, and slower still to grasp the opportunity to enlarge its professional membership pool. Measures to achieve this wider membership were, however, eventually put in place, and I welcome them.

Dangers avoided

One of the risks of seeking changes in an existing Act of Parliament so as to eliminate its identified defects is that the clauses that do not need amendment, because they are appropriate and operating well, may be tampered with. It is not unknown for such damage to occur. Thankfully, the Nurses, Midwives and Health Visitors Act 1979 suffered no such damage, being only improved by the amendments introduced by the 1992 Act. Even though it might not have yet reached perfection, the nursing, midwifery and health visiting professions in the United Kingdom are fortunate in their legislation. Their fellow professionals in many other countries, like the members of some other professions in this country, are, not surprisingly, covetous of that legislation.

To have legislation that opens with the statement that 'The principal functions of the Council shall be to establish and improve standards of training and professional conduct for nurses, midwives and health visitors' is to have a firm foundation on which to build. There is a great deal in that excellent statement in statute law that the professions have yet to explore and exploit.

To have legislation that requires that the Council 'shall, by means of rules (i.e. subordinate legislation) determine the conditions of a person's being admitted to training, and the kind, content and standard of that training to be undertaken with a view to registration' protects the status and significance of registration against dilution.

To have legislation that makes it clear that it is the Council – the profession's regulatory body – that has been given the power of providing, 'in such manner as it thinks fit, advice for nurses, midwives and health visitors on standards of professional conduct' is strength indeed.

To have law that does not impose boundaries around the practice of the persons regulated by the body it has created, but instead allows for a flexible and innovative approach to practice is something to treasure.

Conclusion

It was my privilege, by virtue of the post with the UKCC that I held at the time, to be deeply involved in the preparation and progression of the amendments to the 1979 Act to which I have referred above. The open and cooperative manner in which civil servants joined together with representatives of the regulatory bodies in promoting these improvements made this an enjoyable experience. The positive outcomes amply justified the work involved.

It is now incumbent on the Council, and the associated National Boards in each country of the United Kingdom, to ensure that it uses to the maximum the positive legislation that established them and prescribes their functions.

References

1 *Nurses, Midwives and Health Visitors Act 1979*. London: HMSO.
2 *Nurses, Midwives and Health Visitors Act 1992*. London: HMSO.
3 Robinson J. (1988) A patient voice at the GMC – a lay member's view of the General Medical Council. London: *Health Rights*.

Section III

Professional Regulation in Practice

Chapter 7

Advice, Guidance and Standards

One of the essential elements of professional regulation which I have described in Chapter 2 is that of the advice, guidance and standards that should be provided directly by a regulatory body for the benefit of all its registered practitioners, and through their practice, for the benefit of the public. The response to this takes various forms with different professions and in different countries.

As far as the nursing, midwifery and health visiting professions in the United Kingdom are concerned, the correct note is struck by the legislation (the Nurses, Midwives and Health Visitors Act 1979) which established the regulatory body for these professions. At section 2(1) it states that:

> 'The principal functions of the Central Council shall be to establish and improve standards of training and professional conduct for nurses, midwives and health visitors.'[1]

The reader will note the power of this short sentence. The improvement of standards of conduct by the profession's regulatory body is to be a principal function, and, because the word 'shall' is to be found at the heart of the sentence, it is to be a mandatory function.

Better still, the point is reinforced only four sentences later in the same Act of Parliament when section 2(5) is seen to state that:

> 'The powers of the Council shall include that of providing, in such manner as it thinks fit, advice for nurses, midwives and health visitors on standards of professional conduct.'

So the law can be seen to have prescribed not only one of the outcomes that was to be achieved – improvement in standards of professional conduct – but one of the means by which that is to be achieved – the dissemination of advice by the regulatory body 'in such manner as it thinks fit'. This I regard as a very significant piece of legislation, not least because I take it as meaning that the improvement it requires is not something to be achieved at the outset to arrive at a new 'conduct' plateau, but a perpetual activity.

The regulatory body created by this legislation (the United Kingdom Central Council for Nursing, Midwifery and Health Visiting, or UKCC) to replace a number of previous regulatory bodies, delighted that its authority to provide advice on standards of professional conduct was now unequivocally stated in law, has, since its inception in 1983, responded in a number of ways. Central to its 'advice for nurses, midwives and health visitors' is its *Code of Professional Conduct for the Nurse, Midwife and Health Visitor*, now in its third edition.[2]

The Code of Professional Conduct

On each of the occasions that the UKCC has published a new edition of the Code it has distributed it directly to all those on its register whose registration is current and effective. It has also been made available to organisations that represent the interests of users of the health services, to the regulatory and professional membership organisations for other health professions, and to any private individuals who wish to be aware of its contents.

During the life of the three editions of this Code, it has been the subject of many articles and letters in the professional journals. One of the first to go into print when the first edition was published in 1983 was Annie Altschul. In an article entitled 'Shout at the Minister' she wrote:

> 'The effect on patients of nurses who feel harassed and who know that no matter how hard they work, they are unable to give proper standards of care, has rarely been documented and used as evidence to those who are in positions of power.
>
> The duty to do this is now quite openly laid on every nurse by the United Kingdom Central Council for Nursing, Midwifery and Health Visiting. Every nurse now has in her possession the Code of Professional Conduct.
>
> The duty of every trained nurse is now absolutely clear. She is accountable for her own actions and responsible for the work of her subordinates. If she carries on in spite of being short staffed or inappropriately staffed, without letting those higher in the nursing hierarchy know, she is personally accountable and patients and the public in general should be encouraged to demand that she is held accountable.'[3]

Since publication of the current (third) edition of the Code I have personally published numerous articles to elaborate upon its contents and significance. These have included 'Accountability in Principle and Practice',[4] 'Professional Conduct and Accountability'[5] and 'Empowerment through use of the Code of Professional Conduct'.[6]

The text of the third edition of the Code reads as follows:

> 'Each registered nurse, midwife and health visitor shall act, at all times, in such a manner as to:
>
> - safeguard and promote the interests of individual patients and clients;
> - serve the interests of society;
> - justify public trust and confidence and
> - uphold and enhance the good standing and reputation of the professions.
>
> As a registered nurse, midwife or health visitor, you are personally accountable for your practice and, in the exercise of your professional accountability, must:

1 act always in such a manner as to promote and safeguard the interests and well-being of patients and clients;

2 ensure that no action or omission on your part, or within your sphere of responsibility, is detrimental to the interests, condition or safety of patients and clients;

3 maintain and improve your professional knowledge and competence;

4 acknowledge any limitations in your knowledge and competence and decline any duties or responsibilities unless able to perform them in a safe and skilled manner;

5 work in an open and cooperative manner with patients, clients and their families, foster their independence and recognise and respect their involvement in the planning and delivery of care;

6 work in a collaborative and cooperative manner with health care professionals and others involved in providing care, and recognise and respect their particular contributions within the care team;

7 recognise and respect the uniqueness and dignity of each patient and client, and respond to their need for care, irrespective of their ethnic origin, religious beliefs, personal attributes, the nature of their health problems or any other factor;

8 report to an appropriate person or authority, at the earliest possible time, any conscientious objection which may be relevant to your professional practice;

9 avoid any abuse of your privileged relationship with patients and clients and of the privileged access to their person, property, residence or workplace;

10 protect all confidential information concerning patients and clients obtained in the course of professional practice and make disclosures only with consent, where required by the order of a court or where you can justify disclosure in the wider public interest;

11 report to an appropriate person or authority, having regard to the physical, psychological and social effects on patients and clients, any circumstances in the environment of care which could jeopardise standards of practice;

12 report to an appropriate person or authority any circumstances in which safe and appropriate care for patients and clients cannot be provided;

13 report to an appropriate person or authority where it appears that the health or safety of colleagues is at risk, as such circumstances may compromise standards of practice and care;

14 assist professional colleagues, in the context of your own knowledge, experience and sphere of responsibility, to develop their professional competence, and assist others in the care team, including informal carers, to contribute safely and to a degree appropriate to their roles;

15 refuse any gift, favour or hospitality from patients or clients currently in your

care which might be interpreted as seeking to exert influence to obtain preferential consideration; and

16 ensure that your registration status is not used in the promotion of commercial products or services, declare any financial or other interests in relevant organisations providing such goods or services and ensure that your professional judgement is not influenced by any commercial considerations.'

I contend that this text has improved on the second edition in a number of important ways. The new emphasis on personal accountability that is found in the stem sentence out of which each of the numbered clauses grows and which it completes is important. To state that '*you* are *personally* accountable for your practice' means that there is no such thing as accountability by proxy, no matter who that proxy might be. To state that '*you* are personally accountable for *your* practice' means *all* of your practice. To use the word '*must*' as the link between the stem sentence and the clause means that the Council regards what follows as mandatory and not optional. Indeed, the terminology employed in this 'accountability' stem is making the point that accountability, in professional practice, is not an optional extra, but an integral, essential and unavoidable element of professional practice.

Improvement can also be identified in the wording of clause 3. Here the former leading words 'take every reasonable opportunity to' have been deleted, leaving the practitioner facing a firm requirement, as an aspect of their personal accountability, to 'maintain and improve your professional knowledge and competence'.

The insertion of an additional clause – the new clause 5 – I regard as of the greatest importance. It is worded so as to seek to encourage a style of practice that respects the autonomy of the individual patient and sheds the paternalism that has often blighted nursing practice in the past. The use of the phrase 'foster their independence' is greatly to be welcomed, as is the use for the first time of 'recognise and respect'. The latter phrase, used again in the two clauses that follow, seems to be saying something much more significant than 'take account of' that was a feature of the previous text.

One further change that I suggest is of enormous importance is that now found in clause 7. This has replaced the former clause 6, which fairly modestly asked the practitioner to 'Take account of the customs, values and spiritual beliefs of patients and clients'. It was my personal experience, while holding senior posts at the UKCC concerned with standards and ethics, that this clause was the subject of more criticism and comment than all of the others combined. The new clause 7 is, I suggest, not only more robust through its use of 'recognise and respect', but is about matters that are at the very heart of good practice in nursing. It is essential that practitioners do recognise and respect 'the uniqueness and dignity of each patient'. It is essential that they practise in a manner that is non-judgmental and non-selective, as this clause requires.

To select for emphasis these few passages of text is not to ignore or denigrate the importance of the remainder. I continue to claim for the whole text the three major functions that were described in the second edition of this book.

The Code as an extended definition of 'accountability'

I have already drawn attention to the emphasis placed on the subject of accountability in the stem sentence of the code from which the remainder of the text then flows.

Although the words 'accountable' and 'accountability' each appear only once in the document, because they appear where they do, and because the document is constructed in the way it is, those words appear, in effect, sixteen times. Clause 1 does not begin with the words 'act always in such a manner ...' It begins with 'As a registered nurse, midwife or health visitor, you are personally accountable...'. It seems justifiable, therefore, to argue that the Code of Professional Conduct is, for nurses, midwives and health visitors, an extended definition of accountability. It is that theme of accountability that provides the central focus of a document which promotes the idea that practitioners will conduct themselves in the manner it describes and will do so because it is manifestly in the interests of those they serve.

The Code of Professional Conduct therefore seeks to assist practitioners to come to grips with their personal accountability by providing an important set of principles. It would not be appropriate – indeed it would be impossible – for a regulatory body to say to its practitioners 'In situation X, do this'. Recognising that each practitioner has to make judgments in a wide variety of circumstances and to be answerable – i.e. able to be called to account – for those judgments, it must surely be appropriate, however, for that body to provide a structure within which to exercise such judgment.

This key, though brief, document does not, therefore, seek to say everything that there is to be said in fine detail. One of the things it does, in effect, say, however, is that each and every practitioner who is on the Council's register is expected to set and achieve high standards and thereby to honour the requirements of the code generally and its first clause in particular.

There are those who seek to denigrate the status and importance of codes or professional declarations in general and this one in particular. While I understand some of their arguments, I do not agree with their conclusions. In one conference paper (often repeated, but not published), prepared initially in response to an invitation to address the subject *Professional Standards, Codes and Guidelines: A Help or a Hindrance?*,[7] I have stated my firm conclusion that, on balance, and recognising some of their limitations, they are a significant help.

It is certainly the case that, in preparing and distributing the code on which I am now concentrating, the emphasis of which is the primacy of the patient's interests, and also in publishing documents which promote standards in specific areas of practice, the UKCC is in harmony with a broad and international medical and nursing practice and approach. I have in mind such documents from within my own profession as *The Code for Nurses* published by the International Council of Nurses[8] (which might be regarded as the parent document of the UKCC Code) and the *Code for Nurses with Interpretive Statements* published by the American Nurses Association[9] (which stirred some of the ideas now reflected in the UKCC Code). I think also of some relevant documents from medical organisations within the United Kingdom, including the British Medical Association's *Medical Ethics Today: Its Practice and Philosophy*[10] and the General Medical Council's succinct and excellent *The Duties of a Doctor.*[11] And I note that Downie and Calman, though appearing to be critical of codes for their limitations, still come to the interesting conclusion that 'It is therefore important that professions have codes with which to defend themselves against the wrong kind of political interference'.[12]

It was necessary, and still is necessary, for the UKCC to direct the attention of practitioners to the important subject of accountability and to focus their attention on the things for which they might be called to account. Why not do it, then, in this succinct form? Unfortunately there are still far too many practitioners who have not yet grasped the size and nature of their personal accountability. The message has to be repeated again and again. Some of the cases and studies in Chapters 13 and 14 illustrate this conclusion and seek to make a contribution to remedying the situation by providing discussion material. Bear this definition of the Code of Professional Conduct in mind when you consider them.

The Code as a portrait

I present the Code of Professional Conduct to you as a portrait of the kind of person the UKCC thinks we need and wants to see in the profession. If you examine the Code as a portrait, what do you see? I hope that you find, as I do, that the introductory paragraph provides an answer to the question. It is saying, is it not, that this is the portrait of someone who conducts themselves in such a manner as to justify public trust and confidence, who is keen to serve the interests of society at large, who recognises the importance of upholding and enhancing the good standing and reputation of her or his profession (since without that how can there be public trust and confidence?), but who above all, in a direct sense, acts so as to safeguard and promote the interests of individual patients. The words of the introductory paragraph of the code are no sinecure. They are of value in their own right, but then provide the general foundation on which the whole text is built.

So once again, when you look at the Code as a portrait, what kind of portrait do you see? I hope that you find there a description of a person who is clear about the primacy of the patient's interests – something that is there either overtly or implicitly in every clause. But it is also the portrait of a person who is a professional in her or his own right, both equipped and willing to recognise the direct responsibility that goes with that status. It is also the portrait of a person whose concern for patients means that they will not silently tolerate the intolerable and that they will equip themselves to be articulate in their representations about those things which obstruct the delivery of good care, place patients at risk, jeopardise standards or endanger colleagues. It is a very demanding portrait to match, but that surely does not reduce its significance or appropriateness.

The Code as a template

Another of the Code's important functions is that of providing, for the nurse, midwife or health visitor, a template against which to measure their own conduct, recognising that, should they be the subject of a complaint to the Council that calls into question their registration status, it will be used in the same way by the relevant committee in determining whether the conduct complained of (if proved to the required standard) amounts to misconduct in a professional sense. Enlightened self-interest on the part of the practitioner should therefore guide her or him to recognising the importance of the document and regarding it in this way. It seems entirely reasonable that, having stated its expectations through the Code's text, the Council should use it in this way. It would surely have been unreasonable of the Council, possessing as it does the power to remove a person from the register for misconduct, had it failed to make public its expectations and, therefore, its template.

From within days of the publication of the first edition in 1983 the Council's Professional Conduct Committee has certainly turned to this template, both to aid the members in determining the issue of misconduct, and also in offering firm guidance to those individual respondents with whom they decide to leave the right to practise.

Other advice, guidance and standards

In the United Kingdom, the regulatory body for the nursing, midwifery and health visiting professions (the UKCC), has published a number of other documents to supplement its Code of Professional Conduct. One of these, published in 1996 to replace three previous advisory documents and address a number of additional practice-related issues is entitled *Guidelines for Professional Practice*.[13] The purpose of this booklet, as stated in its preamble, is to 'provide a guide for reflection on the statements within the Code of Professional Conduct'. It then proceeds to focus attention on a range of important issues, including the practitioner's duty of care, advocacy, autonomy, communication, consent, confidentiality and representing concerns about the environment of care. The whole text is reproduced as Appendix 2.

The Council has also published an important document for the benefit of those who are still on the route to the register. This is entitled *A Guide for Students of Nursing and Midwifery*.[14] This introduces students to the Code of Professional Conduct and the approach to professional practice that it encourages.

It has also produced two important documents promoting good standards in specific areas of practice. These are *Standards for the Administration of Medicines*[15] and *Standards for Records and Record Keeping*.[16] These are reproduced as Appendix 3 and 4 respectively.

From all of this it can be seen that, in the United Kingdom, the liberating aspects of the Nurses, Midwives and Health Visitors Act of 1979 have been and continue to be used to advantage. The documents referred to above challenge practitioners, in a quite stark way, to reject the notion that nurses should be compliant and submissive. This needed to be changed, and, to a substantial degree, still needs to be changed. The message presented by the Code, supplemented by the other documents to which I have referred, is that 'good conduct' involves being honest, open, questioning and challenging for no other reason than that these qualities – supplemented, of course, by knowledge, skill and compassion – are those which best serve the interests of patients.

It remains necessary for the profession to have in place a system which can deal effectively with the relatively small percentage of practitioners in whose hands, for whatever reason, the public cannot be safely placed. It is even more important, however, that each and every individual practitioner within the profession responds to the challenge that they maintain and improve their professional knowledge and skill, and also that they enhance their understanding of the ethical principles and values that underpin good professional practice.

I am pleased to note that there is a steadily increasing literature to assist in achieving this objective. A list of further recommended reading is set out at page 261.

References

1 *Nurses, Midwives and Health Visitors Act 1979*. London: HMSO.
2 *Code of Professional Conduct for the Nurse, Midwife and Health Visitor*, Third Edition (1992). London: UKCC.
3 Altschul A. (1983) Shout at the Minister *Nursing Mirror* 5 October 1983.
4 Pyne R. (1992) Accountability in Principle and Practice. *British Journal of Nursing* 1, 6.
5 Pyne R. (1994) Professional Conduct and Accountability. *Modern Midwife* September 1994.
6 Pyne R. (1994) Empowerment through use of the Code of Professional Conduct. *British Journal of Nursing* 3, 12.
7 Pyne R. (1994) *Professional Standards, Codes and Guidelines: A Help or a Hindrance?*. October 1994 (unpublished paper).
8 *Code for Nurses* (1973). Geneva: International Council of Nurses.
9 *Code for Nurses with Interpretive Statements* (1976). American Nurses Association.
10 *Medical Ethics Today: Its Practice and Philosophy* (1993). London: British Medical Association.
11 *The Duties of a Doctor* (1995). London: General Medical Council.
12 Downie R.S. & Calman K.C. (1994). *Healthy Respect*. Oxford: Oxford University Press.
13 *Guidelines for Professional Practice* (1996). London: UKCC.
14 *A Guide for Students of Nursing and Midwifery* (1992). London: UKCC.
15 *Standards for the Administration of Medicines* (1992). London: UKCC.
16 *Standards for Records and Record Keeping* (1993). London: UKCC.

Chapter 8

Investigating and Judging Alleged Misconduct

Introduction

The purpose of the Nurses, Midwives and Health Visitors Act of 1979 is described in its introductory paragraph. This description states that it makes 'new provision with respect to the education, training, regulation and discipline of nurses, midwives and health visitors and the maintenance of a single professional register.'[1]

The wording is, perhaps, unfortunate, in that it might be interpreted as stating that 'regulation' is something separate from control of the route to the register and the maintenance of registration (the education and training components) or the arrangements for possible removal from the register (the discipline component), or indeed maintenance of the professional register. In fact, as has been argued in Chapter 2, 'regulation', in order to be effective, must include these essential elements and certain others. This chapter is concerned with the discipline component of that definition.

The specific allocation of responsibility in law for all of the investigatory and judgmental work that falls under the general heading of 'discipline' is found in section 12 of the same 1979 Act, as now modified by the Nurses, Midwives and Health Visitors Act of 1992.[2] This states that:

'(1) The Central Council shall by rules determine circumstances in which, and the means by which –

(a) a person may, for misconduct or otherwise, be removed from the register or a part of it, whether or not for a specified period;

(b) a person who has been removed from the register or a part of it may be restored to it;

(c) a person's registration in the register or a part of it may be directed to be suspended, that is to say not to have effect during such a period as may be specified in the direction;

(d) the suspension of a person's registration in the register or a part of it may be terminated; and

(e) an entry in the register may be removed, altered or restored.

(2) Committees of the Council shall be constituted by the rules to deal with proceedings for a person's removal from, or restoration to, the register or for the removal, alteration or restoration of any entry.

(3) The committees need not be constituted exclusively from members of the Council, but the rules shall provide, in relation to committees constituted by them, that there shall only be a quorum if a majority of those present are members of the Council.
(4) The rules shall so provide that members of a committee constituted to adjudicate upon the conduct of any person are selected with due regard to the professional field in which that person works.
(5) The rules shall make provision as to the procedure to be followed, and the rules of evidence to be observed, in such proceedings, whether before the Council itself or before any committee so constituted, and for the proceedings to be in public except in such cases (if any) as the rules may specify.
(6) Schedule 3 to this Act has effect with respect to the conduct of proceedings to which this section applies.'

Section 12A supplements that with the following text:

'(1) Without prejudice to the generality of section 12, rules under that section may make provision with respect to the giving, in the course of disciplinary proceedings, of cautions as to future conduct.
(2) Rules under section 12 may also make provision with respect to the keeping by the Council of a record of any caution as to future conduct given in the course of disciplinary proceedings.
(3) For the purposes of this section, "disciplinary proceedings" means proceedings for removal from the register or a part of it for misconduct.'

In passing into law the Nurses, Midwives and Health Visitors Act of 1992 the United Kingdom Government was responding to the pressure for positive change exerted, in the light of experience of operating the 1979 Act since 1983, and to the recommendations of the consultants through whom it conducted its review of that Act in operation. This important new legislation made a number of important changes which enhanced the Council's powers and made it possible for it to operate in a more flexible manner.

The new power of suspension

First among these important changes was the introduction of a power to suspend registration, as distinct from removal from the register. This additional power was sought for two reasons. First, to avoid stigmatising the person who, by decision of the Health Committee (see Chapter 9) was to be prevented from practice because it had been judged that their fitness to practise was seriously impaired by illness. The view had been formed that the decision which prevented them from practising should, wherever appropriate, be different from that applied to those who had been removed as a result of their proven misconduct. 'Suspension' in this form was expected to be applied to Health Committee cases rather than Professional Conduct Committee cases, although it is not limited to the former.

There was, however, a second and very significant benefit to be gained from this new power to 'suspend'. Since the introduction of regulatory procedures for nurses and midwives in the early years of the twentieth century, the bodies concerned had no power to prevent a person on the register from practising while complaints against them were being investigated or while awaiting a hearing before the Professional Conduct Committee. This simple amendment to allow 'suspension' made it possible for the Council to make 'rules' which would address this disturbing problem by introducing 'interim suspension'. The Council's document *Complaints about Professional Conduct*[3] explains its use of this new power in the following terms:

> 'The Committee [i.e. the Preliminary Proceedings Committee] may also consider whether to impose interim suspension of a practitioner's registration, pending further investigation, and/or early referral to the Professional Conduct or Health Committee. This power will only be used, very occasionally, in circumstances where it is clear that, in the interests of public safety, or in the practitioner's own interest, interim suspension should be imposed.'

The power of 'interim suspension', linked to an awareness of the fact that, where this power is used it is incumbent on the Council to complete its investigations and bring the case for full hearing before the Professional Conduct Committee at the earliest possible date, has been well and selectively used. It has clearly enhanced the Council's power to serve and protect the public interest.

Broader membership of committees

Prior to the passing into law of the 1992 Act, committees concerned with disciplinary matters, unlike other Council committees concerned with education and practice matters, had to be composed entirely of persons who were members of the Council. This sometimes created serious problems. Council members, with few exceptions, have demanding full-time jobs. The time demands of the Professional Conduct Committee are enormous. For example, the Professional Conduct Committee (normally five members drawn from the pool) met for 167 days in the year 1995/1996. The new clause made it possible to draw upon two other categories of persons in order to constitute a Professional Conduct Committee.

First, members of the professions who are not Council members. This carried a potential benefit of enlarging the pool from which a committee had to be convened, and helping to satisfy the requirement that the committee that sits in judgment on a respondent practitioner be selected with due regard to the field in which that practitioner worked or had worked. This was impossible to satisfy if the Council membership included nobody from the respondent's sphere of practice. While this did not particularly matter if the case was concerned (for example) with theft of controlled drugs from a ward's stock, it did if the allegations related to some very specific aspects of specialist practice. Surprisingly, given the demands on the time of members and occasional problems in satisfying the 'due regard' criterion, the Council was slow to pass through the door which the 1992 Act and the supplementary rules had made possible, but measures have now been taken to involve other members of the professions that the Council regulates. This was an important development.

So also was the opportunity the new clause provided, and which was grasped more speedily by the Council, to create an additional member pool composed of lay persons nominated for appointment by recognised consumer organisations with an interest in health care. The creation of a pool of this kind made it possible, on almost all occasions, to ensure that the membership of a particular Professional Conduct Committee convened to hear a specific case or cases would include a person who would be able to view the misconduct, if proven, from an intelligent lay or public perspective, as distinct from the professional standpoint. The requirement that, in order to be quorate, a majority of Council members must be members of the particular committee leaves it bearing responsibility for this important area of its work, while broadening the membership in a positive way.

The power of caution

Another major step forward achieved by the amendments contained in the 1992 Act was the introduction of a power to administer formal cautions as to future conduct and for such cautions to remain on a person's record with the Council for a period, able to be cited as relevant antecedent history should the person appear again and be found guilty of misconduct in a professional sense while that record exists.

This was a very important development. Prior to this change in the law the Investigating Committees (the predecessors of the Preliminary Proceedings Committee), if they believed that the allegations against an individual were either proved by criminal conviction or were capable of proof by the available evidence and were likely to be regarded as misconduct, had either to forward a case for hearing before the Professional Conduct Committee or take no action. It was often the view of the members that, although they did not believe that the allegations (often admitted) should lead to removal from the register, to do nothing sent out the wrong message – one that was able to be construed as the committee condoning the unacceptable conduct of the practitioner involved. Many cases were forwarded to the Professional Conduct Committee over the years which contained no serious prospect of removal from the register, but they had to be scheduled and heard in accordance with the required strict rules of evidence. This contributed to a serious delay in getting cases heard, and undoubtedly meant that some practitioners who needed to be removed from the register as an urgent public interest measure were left with the right to practise for disturbingly long periods.

A similar dilemma existed for the Professional Conduct Committee. Previously, where it had proved the facts alleged against a practitioner and determined that those facts were misconduct in a professional sense, after hearing evidence concerning the context of the offence, the practitioner's career record and any mitigation, it had either to remove that practitioner from the register or take no action. In many cases the former decision seemed too harsh in the particular circumstances of the specific case, yet once again the latter seemed to imply that the practitioner's actions or omissions, by now labelled 'professional misconduct', were condoned. The authority which the new law provided to administer a formal caution both strengthened the procedures and made them more logical.

These new powers, sought by the Council and granted by Parliament, have improved the legislation immeasurably.

Statutory rules

Under the terms of that statement of responsibility set out in the Act as now amended, and using the authority which it confers, the Council has prepared the required subordinate legislation (the 'rules'). The Act is the primary legislation – that which is approved directly by Parliament. Rules are the secondary or subordinate legislation which the Council must prepare, having first considered with care the policies it wishes to pursue, the powers it wishes to hold and the procedures it wishes to adopt. In common with comparable statutory regulatory organisations for other professions, the Council can only prepare rules for which a source exists in primary legislation.

The rules that apply to the investigation and judgment of allegations of misconduct at the time of writing are those set out in *Statutory Instrument 1993, No. 893, The Nurses, Midwives and Health Visitors Rules, 1993.*[4] In the case of the rules contained in this statutory instrument, considering the awesome powers which they provide for the Council, the approval has to be gained of the Lord Chancellor (for England and Wales), the Lord Advocate (for Scotland) and the Lord Chief Justice in Northern Ireland.

These statutory rules establish, with considerable precision, how the powers provided by section 12 of the 1979 Act, as now amended by the 1992 Act, are to be used and its requirements satisfied.

In the residue of this chapter I focus attention on the role and function of the committees responsible for the sieving and judgmental stages respectively of the disciplinary process. The reader who requires a fuller explanation of the roles, functions and sources of membership of the United Kingdom Central Council for Nursing, Midwifery and Health Visiting and its related National Boards can refer to the detailed description I have provided in another publication.[5] Suffice it for the purposes of this chapter to state that nurses, midwives and health visitors in current practice form a significant majority of the membership of both the Council and the Boards. The important principle of the profession regulating itself in the public interest is therefore honoured.

Complaints alleging misconduct

The law is written in such a way that it is open to any person to bring to the attention of the Council an allegation that a person on its register has, through something he or she had done or has failed to do, raised questions about their appropriateness to retain that registration status and consequent right to practise. The Council has published (in 1993) a document to assist potential complainants to understand both the system for dealing with allegations of misconduct and those which suggest unfitness to practise due to illness. This document (*Complaints about Professional Conduct*) is reproduced as Appendix 6.

Investigation

The publication mentioned above contains (in its Annexes A and B) a flow diagram which explains, in simplified form, the process by which an allegation of misconduct is considered. From the diagram it can be noted that the complaints which require investigation and subsequent consideration come from two sources.

Findings of guilt in criminal courts

One source of complaint is the criminal courts. Systems exist in each of the four countries of the United Kingdom which seek to ensure that, where a person known or believed to be a registered nurse, midwife or health visitor has been found guilty of a type of offence that may raise questions about his or her future registration status, a formal notification is submitted so that the matter may be given due consideration.

The notification of a finding of guilt having been received, it is then necessary to obtain from the officers of the relevant court a certificate of conviction or a certificate of the adjudication of the court. The effect of section 13 of the Powers of the Criminal Courts Act 1973 is that a 'true conviction' is only deemed to exist if the court, having established guilt through either the defendant's admission or by hearing convincing evidence, then imposes an actual penalty. These take the form of an actual or suspended prison sentence, a monetary fine, a community service order or (in Scotland only) an admonition. If the person, having been found guilty, is then made the subject of an absolute or conditional discharge or a probation order no penalty is deemed to have been imposed by the judicial system. While a notification of the finding of guilt should be submitted where the offence is of a relevant kind, further proceedings cannot be taken by other bodies based on that finding alone. It is necessary to assemble evidence of witnesses to be called should the case be referred for Professional Conduct Committee hearing and the person not admit to the charge or charges.

In those cases where the criminal court hearing has concluded with a 'true conviction' the assembly of evidence is relatively simple. A certificate of conviction from an appropriate officer of the court which heard the case is proof of the facts of which the person was convicted and he or she is not allowed to go behind that conviction. This fact emphasises how essential it is that registered professional practitioners (in any profession) should not plead guilty in court if they are not, since that plea may have profound effects on their professional career.

This illustrates how one section of the law can affect the operation of another. Faced with two nurses who have pleaded guilty to exactly the same offence and who have similar mitigation to offer, one group of magistrates may fine the nurse appearing before them a small sum of money (therefore a true conviction) while another may make their guilty nurse the subject of a probation order. The statutory bodies can deal with both cases, though the second only at greater cost and inconvenience. Provided guilt has been established, it is the offence and not the penalty that determines whether the case should be reported.

In addition to obtaining a formal certificate of conviction, it is usual, in investigating a conviction case, to obtain a statement from a relevant police officer as to the circumstances leading up to the conviction.

The very existence of the reporting system referred to above reinforces the status of nursing, midwifery and health visiting in the United Kingdom. The general (and I believe totally reasonable) philosophy behind this practice is that policemen, magistrates or even judges cannot properly determine what is of concern to a particular profession, but rather that such matters should be considered and determined largely by members of that profession sitting in collective professional judgment.

Other allegations

The second source of reports concerns people on the UKCC's register who have not appeared in court and been found guilty, but whose conduct is perceived by others to be so unsatisfactory as to question seriously their appropriateness to practise, believing vulnerable members of society to be unsafe in their hands.

The majority of such allegations concern incidents occurring in the course of professional practice. They may be by professional or general managers who have already taken a decision to dismiss a practitioner from his or her employment, but who, after consideration, take the view that the conduct that led to that decision also raises serious questions about that person's appropriateness to practise with patients or clients at all. They may be made by professional colleagues (often quite junior and recently qualified colleagues), sometimes only after their own managers have responded in what they regard as an inadequate way to serious complaints taken to them in the interest of patients and supported by clear evidence. They may be brought to the attention of the regulatory body by patients, their relatives or other visitors, or by any individual who feels concerned about something he or she has observed. It is unfortunate, therefore, that, by producing its document entitled *Reporting misconduct – information for employers and managers*,[6] the Council may have reinforced the myth that only those holding such posts can bring complaints which call into question a person's registration status.

It is, then, any person's right to complain about any nurse, midwife or health visitor. Whether that person is a professional manager, a colleague, a patient or someone else, that right in this matter is still the same. It is incumbent on the statutory body, having received a complaint, to investigate it with the same zeal and thoroughness, irrespective of the source.

It must, of course, be the case that no practitioner can have his or her name removed from the register and thus be prevented from practising on the basis of another person's unproven statements and allegations. Those allegations must be thoroughly investigated and tested, no matter what the cost in time or money. It is to assist people in this potential complainant category particularly that the UKCC has published and distributed the document found at Appendix 6.

The formal complaint alleging misconduct is but the beginning of the process. It is then necessary to have the complaint investigated. This will involve identifying those people who were present at the time and place of an alleged incident and can be called to give evidence should the case be referred for professional conduct hearing. This stage of assembly of the evidence is very important. Statements must be obtained from those who will be or may be called in evidence, it being recognised that the standard of evidence is that of the criminal courts and not the much lesser standard (giving credence to hearsay evidence, etc.) of employment disciplinary proceedings.

The practitioner's statement

It is essential, of course, to obtain both sides of any story. Therefore, as well as assembling all the available evidence in support of allegations against a practitioner, the written response of that practitioner to the allegations is sought. The process is the same where there has been a conviction. These documents together form the material which will be considered by the Preliminary Proceedings Committee.

The Preliminary Proceedings

As the flow diagram in Annexe A of Appendix 6 indicates, the Preliminary Proceedings Committee has three options from which to choose. A number of the statutory body's members who have accepted the onerous responsibility of serving on the Preliminary Proceedings Committee will have considered the papers individually in advance. They now assemble to convert their individual reactions to the information before them into a collective professional judgment.

Unlike their predecessors with the former statutory bodies prior to July 1983, if they see evidence that the conduct that has resulted in an allegation of misconduct may be indicative or symptomatic of illness, they can decide to direct the case into a more appropriate channel, where the health of the practitioner can be considered. (That system is the subject of Chapter 9.) If the view is taken that the problem is one of conduct rather than illness, three choices remain.

If the members believe either that there is insufficient evidence to prove the allegations against a named practitioner, or that (even if proved) the facts are not such as to warrant removal of the practitioner's name from the professional register, a decision to close the case will be made and no further action will be taken in respect of those allegations. If, on the other hand, the members believe that there is evidence to substantiate the allegations and that, if proved, removal from the register must be regarded as a distinct possibility, the case will be referred for a hearing before the Professional Conduct Committee. In addition, since 1993 the Committee has the additional power to administer, in writing, a formal caution, but this can only be done if the facts alleged have been admitted and the practitioner has indicated a willingness to accept that those facts amount to misconduct in a professional sense. The practitioner will be advised, in writing, after the Preliminary Proceedings Committee consideration of the case, which of the decisions has been made. Since 1993 the committee's powers also include that of ordering immediate interim suspension of a practitioner's registration. A brief description of this power and the circumstances in which it is used has been provided earlier in this chapter.

The notice of inquiry

There can be very few letters received by any practitioner which match in significance that which formally notifies him or her of the hearing which might culminate in removal from the register. The statutory rules prescribe the wording of the letter into which the specific charges and information as to time and place are inserted. This states:

> 'Take notice that the charge(s) against you, particulars of which are set forth below, has(have) been brought to the notice of the Council, and that the Professional

Conduct Committee of the Council proposes to investigate such charge(s) at a meeting to be held at ... and to determine whether your name should be removed from the register or any part or parts of it.

You are hereby required to attend before the Professional Conduct Committee of the Council at the time and place mentioned above and to answer such charge(s), bringing with you all papers and documents in your possession relevant to the matter and any persons whose evidence you wish to lay before the Professional Conduct Committee.

It should be carefully noted:

You are entitled to be represented at the hearing before the Professional Conduct Committee by a friend (including a spouse or other relative), or by counsel or a solicitor, or by any officer of a professional organisation or trades union, but if you propose to be so represented, you should give written notice to the Registrar of the Council at the address mentioned above at least seven days before the Hearing.'

With this letter the respondent practitioner receives a copy of the current statutory rules which set out in detail the procedures that will be followed in the hearing and the legal disciplines and constraints that apply.

Before that letter is sent the practitioner who is to become the respondent in the case (and their chosen representative if formal notification has been given that there is one) will have received other communications. First, he or she will have received a letter advising that the case has been referred for a hearing. Second, if it is a case other than a true conviction, copies of the statements of the witnesses who are to be called to give evidence are sent so that the respondent is made fully aware of the case he or she has to defend. Third, the respondent is sent a copy of the evidence which has been assembled about his or her previous history and which it is intended be called and submitted only if both the facts alleged and misconduct are proved to the required standard.

The Professional Conduct Committee hearing

Since one of the major purposes of professional regulation is that the interests of the public must be protected from unsafe practitioners, this must be particularly the case with hearings before the Professional Conduct Committee.

It is in recognition of this fact that the Committee meets in public. This makes it possible for members of the public to attend, observe and form a view as to whether the profession is regulating itself in such a manner as to serve the public interest. Access of this kind is facilitated by the Committee meeting not only at its London headquarters but also in venues around the United Kingdom dependent on the geographical distribution of cases.

Although the principal purpose of the public hearing is that stated above, it serves an important secondary purpose. Many members of the profession choose to attend as observers. With few exceptions they report it as being a salutary learning experience which sends them back to their own workplace with their eyes newly opened to some of the hazards they had previously accepted without question.

The Professional Conduct Committee convened for the hearing of a case is made up of five members, a majority of whom must be members of the Council, selected (as the law requires) with due regard to the practitioner's professional field.

The stages of the hearing

There are four specific and separate stages of a hearing which follow the formal reading of the charges and a plea in response. The first is concerned with establishing whether that which is alleged to have happened can be proved. The second is to determine whether any facts which have been established constitute misconduct in a professional sense. The third is to receive evidence about the previous history of the respondent and for him or her to offer evidence in mitigation. The flow diagram (see Annexe B of Appendix 6) indicates the sequence of events but cannot contain explanations of a number of important points.

In the third 'Did it happen?' stage, the standard of evidence is that applying in criminal courts. That is to say that only direct evidence is regarded as admissible and hearsay or second-hand evidence is not. It also means that it is not permitted for either a representative or the Council's solicitor to ask the witnesses leading questions, i.e. questions which imply the answer. This may sometimes result in an allegation that was found proved in a disciplinary hearing of a health authority not being proved before the committee. A legal assessor (a barrister, advocate or solicitor of at least 10 years standing) sits with the Committee to ensure that the rules concerning admissibility of evidence and other matters of law are observed, but does not participate in the decision-making.

Another important point, which is not made apparent in *Complaints about Professional Conduct*, is that the Council has the power to subpoena witnesses and thus compel their attendance. It is unfortunate that the document produced by the Council to supplement it (*Reporting misconduct – information for employers and managers*) omits to mention this important power, and implies by this omission that unless the witnesses to an incident are willing to attend a hearing, it cannot proceed.

Just as the standard of evidence is strict, so also is the standard of proof. It is not sufficient that the committee members think that the matters alleged probably happened. In order to find the facts alleged in any charge proved, the members must be satisfied to the degree of being sure. Mere probability will not suffice. No lesser standard would be acceptable when the Committee has in its power a sanction as enormous as that of removing a person's right to practise in his or her chosen profession.

If the facts alleged in one or more charges against a respondent are proved to the required standard, the committee must then decide whether those facts are to be regarded as misconduct in a professional sense. Before doing so the respondent or representative is given further opportunity to address the Committee and to call further evidence. The Council's solicitor is unlikely to call further evidence, recognising that the case is being heard by a committee that has the relevant expertise within its membership. In deciding whether the facts are to be regarded as misconduct in a professional sense, the Committee will consider those facts in the context of their occurrence rather than in isolation. The members will also have regard to the advice given by the Council regarding expected standards of conduct (in its Code of

Professional Conduct) and to the definition of misconduct in the Professional Conduct Rules. The latter states that 'Misconduct is conduct unworthy of a nurse, midwife or health visitor'.

If misconduct is proved in respect of any of the charges, the Committee must then receive information concerning the respondent's previous history. The Council's solicitor, through evidence or other assembled material, will provide factual information concerning any previous criminal convictions, findings of misconduct or formal disciplinary action.

The respondent can then submit any evidence in mitigation he or she has assembled. This may take the form of further witnesses called to testify as to the respondent's character or written documents.

Only when all of that is completed will the committee retire, to consider in private which of the judgments available to it is appropriate to the case.

Passing judgment

As with the Preliminary Proceedings Committee, the Professional Conduct Committee, if it takes the view that the matters before it are or may be a product of illness, can transfer the case into the other channel which will consider medical evidence (see Chapter 9). If that course of action is not taken there are four options from which the members of the Professional Conduct Committee can choose.

Postponement of judgment

Ultimately the respondent practitioner's name must either be removed from the register or not be removed. The law provides another, essentially interim solution which is to postpone its judgment on the misconduct the committee has had proved to its satisfaction.

If the Committee decides to postpone its judgment it means that the respondent's name remains on the register and that he or she can apply for or hold any post for which the relevant qualifications are held. It also means, however, that the person must appear again before a committee which still has the option of removal from the register to use if it deems it necessary in the public interest. Therefore, in announcing a decision to postpone judgment in a case, the Committee chairman must also indicate the period of postponement and any criteria that the members wish to see satisfied during that period.

At a resumed hearing the Committee, again meeting in public, is presented with information concerning the facts that were established and found to be misconduct in a professional sense. References from persons nominated by the respondent are also received. The law requires that the persons nominated as referees must be aware of the facts previously established and must have known the respondent practitioner during the period of postponement. Reports (e.g. from the Nurses' Welfare Service, probation officers, etc.) are also received. On the basis of all of this information the Committee members then question the practitioner before allowing him or her a final opportunity to address them in further mitigation. The Committee then retires to arrive at its decision.

Postponed judgment decisions have become quite rare since the committee was granted the power, in appropriate cases, to administer formal cautions.

Removal from the professional register

At either a first hearing or a hearing resumed at the end of a period of postponed judgment, the Professional Conduct Committee has the same options from which to choose. If postponement of judgment is discarded the Committee, meeting in private, next considers whether to remove the respondent's name from the Council's register. If it so decides, the decision is immediately effective. A decision to remove a practitioner's name from the register is never taken lightly. It is an enormous sanction. The person has been admitted to the room as a registered nurse, midwife or health visitor, or possessed of registration in more than one such category, and now leaves the room no longer possessed of that status. The making of such a decision is an uncomfortable burden to bear, but the members recognise that, at the point of making it, they act on behalf of the entire registered profession and with the interests of the vulnerable public to the fore.

Formal caution

Where the Committee is satisfied that the facts alleged have been proved to the required standard and have deemed those facts to be misconduct, but has chosen neither to postpone judgment nor to remove from the register, it must next consider whether to use its power to administer a caution. This is a significant sanction since, if taken, that caution remains on the practitioner's registration entry for 5 years and will be made known to any person who seek's confirmation of her or his registration status.

Misconduct proved but no further action

If the Committee rejects the postponed judgment option and decides that the proved misconduct, when considered in context and in the light of the respondent's previous history and general character, does not necessitate removal from the register or the administration of a formal caution, the case is closed. That should not be regarded as an indication that the Committee condones or regards as acceptable the actions or omissions it has both proved and regarded as misconduct. Nor should it be interpreted as an indication that the respondent has been, in any way, 'let off'. He or she, in a public hearing, has been found guilty of misconduct in a professional sense by a committee of his or her peers. That finding will be held on record for 5 years and will be brought forward as important antecedent history if, at any time within that period, the practitioner is found guilty of further misconduct.

Announcement of the committee's judgment

The wording of the statutory rule governing the announcement of the Committee's decision requires that the chairman announce the decision in whatever terms the committee determines. This passage of subordinate law is extremely important, since it means not only that (whatever decision has been made) a public comment can be made about the respondent practitioner's conduct, but comment can also be passed concerning the setting in which the incident(s) occurred, where that is appropriate. This can often serve to make an apparently surprising decision not to remove a person's name completely understandable.

Appeal against removal

Given the enormity of the ultimate sanction available to the Professional Conduct Committee, it is neither surprising nor unreasonable that section 13 of the Nurses, Midwives and Health Visitors Act 1979 allows that 'A person aggrieved by a decision to remove him from the register ... may, within 3 months after the date on which notice of the decision is given to him by the Council, appeal to the appropriate court...'.

The UKCC, like the statutory regulatory bodies for other professions, has found its decisions challenged in the courts more frequently than was the experience of the former statutory bodies. It should not be assumed from that statement that it is a common occurrence, but nine cases in 6 years is a high rate compared with the two appeals against the decisions of the former General Nursing Council (for England and Wales) Disciplinary Committee in its 64 years of existence. The increase in the number of appeals would appear to be a product in part of the greatly increased number of cases being heard, but it is clear that it is also an indication that society at large adopts a more challenging attitude to bodies on which Parliament has conferred substantial powers.

Judicial review

It is not only through appeals tabled under the terms of section 13 of the Act that the courts have become involved in examining specific cases heard by the UKCC's Professional Conduct Committee. Judicial review is a growing area of law and has been used by a small number of practitioners to obtain a review by a judge or judges of a hearing in which, though not removed from the register, the matters alleged against them were proved and regarded as misconduct. This process was also used, with success, in 1996/1997, by a major professional nursing membership organisation to challenge a decision of the Professional Conduct Committee to restore to the register a person it had previously removed for serious criminal offences.

In a minority of the relatively small number of appeal or judicial review cases, those bringing the case have succeeded in having the finding against them set aside. Whatever the outcome, a critical reading of the verbatim transcript of the case by the judges, supplemented by the kind of question and answer process that is a feature of such hearings, has aided a review and some revision of both the committee procedures and statutory rules. For example, different legal assessors took a different view of what might be regarded as admissible under the requirement on the Council's solicitor to present 'evidence as to the previous history of the respondent'. Two appeal cases in which it was alleged that prejudicial material was admitted at that stage served to clarify the matter. This does not necessarily occur, since on some other matters the view presented by the judges in one case has been significantly different from that presented on the same issue by other judges in a second case. It is clear, however, that the judges do not lightly interfere with the decision of a professional committee charged with the onerous burden of considering cases brought against members of their profession without good reason.

Restoration

Removal from the register is not necessarily the end of a person's career as a registered nurse, midwife or health visitor. Indeed, for some it appears to mark the beginning of a necessary professional rehabilitation, the need for which was only recognised when the removal decision was announced.

Section 12(1)(c) of the Nurses, Midwives and Health Visitors Act 1979 provides the basis in primary law for restoration to the register as well as removal from the register.

A person whose name has been removed from the register may make application for restoration as and when he or she so decides. Arrangements then have to be made to hear and consider the application before the Professional Conduct Committee. Before that can take place, references in support of the application must be obtained from persons nominated for that purpose by the applicant. The procedure at the hearing is similar to that described for hearings resumed at the end of a period of postponed judgment. The committee must simply either accept or reject the application. This is an onerous burden for the members, but one from which they must not flinch. In the view of many, this author included, a decision to restore a person to the register is an even bigger decision than that to remove them at an earlier stage. The precedent of the use of the judicial review process having been established to successfully challenge a decision to restore a previously removed person, the Committee must ensure that they do not regard the hearing of restoration applications as of less significance than that to consider allegations with a view to removal.

The workload

The Professional Conduct Committee work makes very large demands upon the members of the Council and others who participate. In the five-year period from 1990/1991 to 1995/1996 the Committee met for 652 full days – an average of 130 days a year. In the course of those years it considered 799 new cases referred by the Preliminary Proceedings Committee, with a view to removal from the register. These meetings have been held in public and at venues throughout the United Kingdom. This has made it possible for both members of the public and the professions regulated by the Council to see this important aspect of the regulatory process in operation.

In 1995/1996 alone, it met on 167 days and heard 127 new cases. In respect of the respondents in these cases, the Committee decided that removal from the register was the appropriate judgment in 73 cases. Of the remainder who were found guilty of misconduct, 32 were the subject of formal caution, judgment was postponed in 1 case, no action was taken in 9 cases and 1 person was referred to the Health Committee. The facts alleged were either not proved or not deemed to amount to professional misconduct in the other cases heard.

During the same one-year period, 24 applications for restoration to the register were considered, of which 14 were accepted and 10 rejected.

Further statistical information concerning this area of the Council's work can be derived from its annual statistical analysis.[7]

A number of Professional Conduct Committee case studies, describing cases that have been heard by the committee, are set out in Chapter 13 of this book for purposes of both information and education. In order to challenge the professional reader, whether from the professions regulated by the Council or another registered health profession, the chapter is deliberately entitled 'Could This Happen Where You Work?'.

Issues arising from professional conduct complaints

In November 1996 the UKCC published an informative and helpful document entitled *Issues arising from professional conduct complaints.*[8] Having first outlined the powers and procedures described in this chapter, it focuses attention on a range of issues emerging from the cases heard over a period of some years which, it contends, have important implications for professional practice.

In particular, it draws attention to issues which managers need to address, particularly concerning management of staff, support for staff, inadequacy of preparation for practice in highly specialised areas and inappropriate delegation to unqualified staff. Seeking to obtain positive advantage and patient-focused improvements from this ostensibly negative aspect of regulatory activity, the document posits an 'Agenda for Action', the bulk of which is directed at managers of health-care facilities and services, but all of which deserves serious consideration by the profession at large.

References

1 *Nurses, Midwives and Health Visitors Act 1979*. London: HMSO.
2 *Nurses, Midwives and Health Visitors Act 1992*. London: HMSO.
3 *Complaints about Professional Conduct* (1993). London: UKCC.
4 *Statutory Instrument 1993, No. 893, The Nurses, Midwives and Health Visitors Rules, 1993*. London: HMSO.
5 Pyne R.H. (1995) The Professional Dimension. In *Nursing Law and Ethics*, edited by J. Tingle & A. Cribb. Oxford: Blackwell Science.
6 *Reporting misconduct – information for employers and managers* (1996). London: UKCC.
7 *Statistical Analysis of the Council's Professional Register, April 1995 to March 1996, Vol. 5* (1996). London: UKCC.
8 *Issues arising from professional conduct complaints* (1996). London: UKCC.

Chapter 9

Investigating and Judging Alleged Unfitness to Practise due to Illness

Introduction

In the early paragraphs of the previous chapter the words of section 12 of the Nurses, Midwives and Health Visitors Act 1979 were drawn to the attention of the reader. It is that passage of the primary law that allows subordinate law ('rules') to be made concerning the circumstances in which and means by which a person may be removed from the professional register.

There is one significant respect in which this passage in present law differs from the comparable passage in the law that established the former statutory bodies (for nursing and midwifery) and governed their proceedings. The old and now repealed laws referred only to establishing rules whereby 'a person may, for misconduct, be removed from the register'. The British Parliament, in its wisdom, replaced this with a passage which refers instead to removal from the register 'for misconduct or otherwise'. The Nurses, Midwives and Health Visitors Act 1992 introduced a further change to allow for not only removal from the register, but also the subtly different 'suspension' from the register. This was deemed important, particularly in respect of persons who needed to be prevented from practising, but were guilty of no culpable action.

The former change was welcomed by those previously involved in operating the law concerning the regulation of nursing and midwifery. All too often they had found themselves in possession of reports about practitioners who were clearly dangerous but about whom they could do nothing since those practitioners, though manifestly unsafe, had done nothing culpable which might be construed as 'misconduct'. All too often, sometimes after incidents with serious or even tragic consequences, they had found themselves using the awesome power of the statutory body's disciplinary machine and a public hearing to deal with someone whose basic problem was their illness.

It had been noted that the 1978 Medical Act had conferred on the General Medical Council not simply a power to consider cases in which it was believed that the fitness to practise of a medical practitioner was seriously impaired by illness but a requirement that it establish and operate the necessary committees and procedures. It was laid out in considerable detail in the primary legislation.

The General Nursing Council for England and Wales, being the statutory body then existing for much the largest number of registered practitioners of nursing, midwifery and health visiting, and consequently having the biggest Disciplinary

Committee caseload, pressed for similar powers, but indicated its preference for a clause in the forthcoming Bill which would simply be enabling in nature and provide for maximum flexibility in subsequent rule-making.

That request for flexibility was satisfied beyond expectations by the simple inclusion of the words 'or otherwise' after 'misconduct' in the clause concerning removal from the register. Those two new words were to prove quite sufficient as a hook in primary legislation on to which the new Council could hang a new set of rules and procedures. It would, as hoped, be possible to enhance the protection afforded the public by allowing the Council to consider reports suggesting that certain practitioners were unfit to practise due to illness.

Sampling the profession's opinion

It was clear, therefore, that the largest of the statutory bodies soon to be replaced had formed the view that a system to protect the public from the practitioner who was unsafe due to illness was necessary. What did the new body (the UKCC) think? Would it choose to use the flexibility provided for it by the Nurses, Midwives and Health Visitors Act 1979?

During the shadow period in which the old and the new bodies overlapped (the old continuing to run things while the new prepared for the future) the UKCC, through one of its working groups convened to examine specific aspects of the new Act, decided that the opportunity provided for it should be grasped. It put this matter as a suggestion to members of the profession through a widely circulated consultation document and found that it received wide support. As a result, the subordinate legislation was prepared and an entirely new aspect of professional regulation came into operation in 1984.

As with the procedures for dealing with allegations of misconduct, those for considering alleged unfitness due to illness are explained in the document *Complaints about Professional Conduct*[1] which is reproduced as Appendix 6. Annexe C of that appendix provides a flow diagram to illustrate, in simplified form, the process by which such complaints or expressions of concern are considered.

Referral from Preliminary Proceedings Committee or Professional Conduct Committee

It has already been explained that if, at any stage of their proceedings, the Preliminary Proceedings Committee or Professional Conduct Committee form the view that the practitioner whose case they are considering is one whose fitness to practise is seriously impaired by illness, they may transfer the case in order that this view be tested through medical examinations and subsequent consideration by the Health Committee.

Direct referral cases

Just as any person has the right to allege that a person on the Council's register is guilty of misconduct in a professional sense and have that thoroughly investigated and competently judged, so also may any person express concern that a practitioner's fitness to practise is seriously impaired by illness and to the danger of his or her patients or clients. These are known as direct referral cases.

Such cases begin with a letter from a concerned individual to the UKCC. That individual will often be a fellow nurse, midwife or health visitor in a management position, but may equally well be a colleague or a private individual. A case of this kind is only formally opened when that original expression of concern is given formal legal status in the form of a statutory declaration. The Council's solicitor therefore takes the original communication and any documents which accompanied it, prepares the statutory declaration and conveys it to the originator to sign if its contents are agreed. The purpose of this procedure is to ensure that the person initiating the case is mindful of the serious nature of the proceedings and the fact that the outcome might be the removal of the practitioner indicated from the professional register. Assistance for employers and managers of nurses about making direct referrals has been provided by the Council in its leaflet *Reporting unfitness to practise – information for employers and managers*.[2] The text is helpful, but the title is unfortunate, since it has to be remembered that any person can make a direct referral, just as they can allege misconduct, and the leaflet contains nothing that is not equally applicable to those who are not managers or employers, but have cause to be concerned about an individual's fitness to practise. It might be construed as meaning that only 'employers and managers' can make such referrals, but this is not the position in law.

The Panel of Professional Screeners

As the flow diagram indicates, such referred cases, once the necessary documentation has been assembled, are referred to a group of UKCC members known as the Panel of Professional Screeners.

Once the screeners have made their decision, the practitioner who is the subject of a case is advised that the referral has been made and invited to undergo medical examination by two of the Council's specifically appointed examiners and at the Council's expense. There is no compulsion on the practitioner to accept that invitation, but if he or she refuses it needs to be recognised that the Health Committee members before whom a hearing will be conducted may infer something from that refusal.

Experience since these procedures came into operation has shown that a majority of practitioners referred by either of the committees in the professional conduct channel accept the invitation and attend for medical examinations.

The role of the screeners is very important. When the members first consider the available material (i.e. the statutory declaration and other annexed documents in a direct referral case, or the documents that were before either the Preliminary Proceedings Committee or Professional Conduct Committee) they must take a view as to whether there is *prima facie* evidence of impairment of fitness to practise through illness. If they decide that there is not, they will close the case if it was a direct referral, or refer it back to the Preliminary Proceedings Committee or Professional Conduct Committee if that was its source.

If they conclude that there is *prima facie* evidence of impairment, they will select the examiners by whom they wish the practitioners to be examined. Assuming the practitioner agrees to examination, the panel of screeners consider the case again with the benefit of the medical reports. At this stage the members must decide either that fitness does appear to be seriously impaired, in which case they refer the case to the Health Committee, or that it is not. In the latter circumstances, as at the previous stage, they either close the case or refer it back to the relevant committee to consider the alleged misconduct. Where the practitioner does not accept the invitation to medical examinations, the screeners have to review the available material again without the benefit of independent medical opinion and make what they believe to be the appropriate decision.

Medical examiners

The medical examiners who serve the Council and the public interest are appointed in accordance with arrangements established by a Schedule of the Professional Conduct Rules. This section of legislation prescribes and lists the medical organisations authorised to nominate specialist registered medical examiners with a view to appointment by the Council. These, in summary, are the various medical Royal Colleges and certain committees of the British Medical Association.

When the nurse, midwife or health visitor referred to the Health Committee in the way described accepts the invitation to medical examinations, arrangements are then made for him or her to be seen by appropriate types of specialists as determined by the screeners. They will be examiners who are remote from both the practitioner's domestic or work settings to ensure an objective approach. To assist them, however, reports will be obtained in advance from the person's general practitioner and any specialist by whom he or she has previously been treated, provided that consent is given for this to be done.

The practitioner's option

The medical examiners submit very detailed medical reports to the relevant UKCC staff. Copies of the reports are then sent to the practitioner about whom they have been written so that he or she is fully aware of the contents of what will be the key documents before the Health Committee. It is then open to the practitioner to decide whether, either with the support of a professional organisation, trades union or other professional adviser, or as a personal decision, to commission one or more further reports from specialists of their own choosing. Sufficient time is allowed both for consideration of this matter and for any further medical examinations to be concluded and the resulting reports prepared and submitted.

As a result of this activity it becomes possible, well in advance of an actual Health Committee hearing, to prepare and circulate a comprehensive document. In the case of a person referred from the Preliminary Proceedings Committee or Professional Conduct Committee, in addition to all the medical reports assembled, any relevant material that was before the referring committee will be included since this may provide some evidence of what might be called symptomatic behaviour.

Since the actual Health Committee hearing is conducted in accordance with the same legally determined procedures irrespective of the source of the referral, I will defer any explanation of it until I have first provided information about the other category of cases – those known as 'direct referral' cases. I do so because there are some significant differences in the procedures that precede the Health Committee hearing.

The Health Committee

As is the case with proceedings before the Professional Conduct Committee, those applying for the Health Committee are set out in detail in Statutory Instrument 1993 No. 893, the title of which is The Nurses, Midwives and Health Visitors (Professional Conduct) Rules, 1993. There are a number of significant differences which it is important to note before considering how the committee is composed and operates.

The pool of members from which, under current law, any particular Health Committee is convened is made up of those members of the Council who do not serve on the Preliminary Proceedings Committee or Panel of Screeners. From these members a committee of five is assembled, the quorum below which the number cannot fall being three members. As with the Professional Conduct Committee, every attempt is made to pay due regard to the practitioner's field of work in assembling a committee.

Hearings in private

Unlike the Professional Conduct Committee, the Health Committee meets in private. The ultimate function of both committees is the protection of the public. It is argued by some that, this being the case, the public should have equal access to both hearings in order to be satisfied about the manner in which the Council exercises its regulatory authority. While being mindful of that argument, the Council, in exercising its rule-making authority, decided that hearings should be in private since the evidence to be received was not that of alleged culpable behaviour but the fine detail of a person's medical history and reports on their current condition. The view was taken that to have public meetings of the Health Committee would inevitably result in breach of confidentiality and would run counter to the rehabilitative influence the Committee might often exert on those appearing before it. This view was seen to be justified in the early years of the Committee's operation, as the rehabilitative influence it hoped to exert often became a reality.

The fact that the meetings are held in private renders the role of the legal assessor even more important. His or her role is to advise the Committee on the admissibility of evidence and matters of law in circumstances in which no public or press comment on the conduct of the case can ever be possible.

The medical examiner role

The statutory rules that govern the Health Committee proceedings require that at least one of the Council's medical examiners who has examined the practitioner and prepared a report must attend to answer questions from that practitioner (or representative) and the Committee and to act as a medical adviser in respect of other information or evidence that emerges in the course of a hearing. If the practitioner so requires, both of the Council examiners involved will attend. Where the practitioner has declined the invitation to undergo medical examinations by Council examiners, one of those who would have been used attends the hearing in the role of medical adviser.

Preparing for the hearing

It is regarded as a matter of great importance that, well before the hearing, the practitioner is sent copies of the entire set of documents that will be before the Committee, when it hears that person's case. This enables him or her, either personally or by taking advice from a professional organisation, trade union, friend or legal adviser, to decide whether to allow the hearing to proceed on the basis of the documentary evidence and medical reports or to require the attendance of relevant people to give oral evidence. With only a small number of exceptions the practitioners, recognising that the medical reports are the most important documents in the set, decide that they do not require the attendance of witnesses. Those who do are often the subject of direct referral cases and have not agreed to be examined by Council examiners.

The hearing

In those cases where oral evidence is required the proceedings are broadly similar to those of the Professional Conduct Committee. That is to say that each witness is questioned first by the person calling him or her (i.e. the Council's solicitor or the practitioner/representative), is then cross-examined and finally questioned by the Committee. The difference lies in the fact that what the Committee must determine, having heard evidence of the symptomatic behaviour giving rise to the complaint, is whether the practitioner's fitness to practise is seriously impaired by illness or not.

In the other cases (where oral evidence is not required) the hearing is based around the assembled documents. In cases referred by one of the committees in the professional conduct channel these will include, in addition to the medical reports, the documents which were before that committee. In direct referral cases the statutory declaration recording the expression of opinion that a practitioner may be unfit to practise, together with any appended witness statements, is included.

Every attempt is made to keep hearings of this kind as informal as is possible and consistent with the fact that, at its conclusion, those who make up the Committee may announce a decision to remove the practitioner's name from the register.

After introductions have been effected, the Committee's chairman formally draws attention to what the statutory rules call 'The grounds for belief that the practitioner's fitness to practise may be seriously impaired by a physical or mental condition'. That done, the attending medical examiner draws attention to points of particular significance in the medical reports and then responds to questions about those reports from the practitioner (or representative) and the Committee.

The practitioner is then questioned by the Committee members. If the practitioner is assisted by the attendance of his or her own medical adviser, that person is then able to address the Committee and answer the members' questions. The attending medical examiner, now cast in the role of medical adviser, is then requested to advise the Committee about any points of significance identified in the course of the proceedings. Finally, the practitioner or representative addresses the Committee before it retires to make its decision.

Committee decision

The Committee must choose from a range of four decisions. At one extreme it can decide that the practitioner's fitness to practise is seriously impaired by illness. If it so decides it must remove or, in the alternative, suspend the practitioner's name from the register, either of which have the effect of preventing the person from practising as a registered nurse, midwife or health visitor. No matter how sympathetic the members may feel towards the practitioner, this is the action the law requires be taken in the public interest.

At the other extreme the Committee can decide that the practitioner's fitness to practise is not seriously impaired by illness. The use of the present tense in the previous sentence is significant. It may well emerge that the practitioner's fitness was seriously impaired at some time in the past and that such impairment led to the actions which became the subject either of allegations of misconduct to the Preliminary Proceedings Committee or direct referral. If the Health Committee decides that the practitioner's fitness to practise is not (definitely) seriously impaired by illness it must close the case. In a small number of cases referred by either the Preliminary Proceedings Committee or the Professional Conduct Committee it emerges that no evidence of illness at the time of the actions or omissions that resulted in allegations of misconduct and which might explain them can be found. In these cases the Health Committee will refer the case back to the Committee whence it came for the 'misconduct' issue to continue to be addressed. It cannot refer to either of those committees a case which began as a direct referral.

Between those extremes the Committee can either postpone its judgment for a stated period or adjourn the hearing for further medical reports. When it takes the former course of action it must indicate the medical evidence it will require for the resumed hearing. When it takes the latter decision it is often because the available medical evidence is contradictory, ambivalent or ambiguous. In such a case the hearing can be resumed as soon as the further medical evidence becomes available. At the resumed hearing of either type of case the procedures are similar to those at the original hearing.

Right of appeal and application for restoration or lifting of suspension

The right to appeal to the relevant court which has been explained in Chapter 8 also applies to the person aggrieved by a 'removal' decision of the Health Committee. So also does the right to apply for restoration to the register. In the latter case the Health Committee hearing the restoration application will require the medical reports specified by the Committee which ordered removal. If satisfied from the medical evidence that the person is again fit to practise, he or she will be restored to the register.

The system is justified

The architects of the Panel of Professional Screeners and Health Committee system have good reason to be pleased with what has been achieved. The protection afforded to the public has undoubtedly been enhanced. In addition to that, a sensitive system now exists which has had a profound rehabilitative effect on the lives of a substantial number of practitioners and will surely continue to do so in respect of other practitioners in the future.

The Nurses, Midwives and Health Visitors Act of 1979 established the United Kingdom Central Council for Nursing, Midwifery and Health Visiting and opened the door for it to introduce this important extension to the regulatory system. Since the Council chose to pass through that door, make the required statutory rules and bring into operation the procedures described above there has been a marked consistency about the types of cases received and considered. A majority of cases each year have been persons with alcohol-related illness. Next come other forms of drug dependence and various manifestations of psychiatric illness.

Statistical information

After doing so in the early years of the operation of the Panel of Screeners and the Health Committee, the Council has ceased to publish even limited statistical information about this important aspect of its work. This is unfortunate and unhelpful, since it conceals, for example, such important information as the number of persons whose registration it finds it necessary to suspend or remove, in the public interest, because of alcohol or drug dependence. Public confidence in the profession is more likely to be enhanced by openness than secrecy, and there seems to be no risk or danger in providing limited statistical data.

References

1 *Complaints about Professional Conduct* (1993). London: UKCC.
2 *Reporting unfitness to practise – information for employers and managers* (1996). London: UKCC.

Chapter 10

The Role of the Nurses Welfare Service

The existence of a welfare or support service linked to the disciplinary function of a statutory body, though still questioned by some practitioners, is now broadly accepted. The suggestion that such a step should be taken was viewed with considerable scepticism when it was first mooted in 1972. In spite of the reservations of many people at that time, the dream of a dedicated few became a reality later in the same year when the former General Nursing Council for England and Wales became the first regulatory body for any of the registered professions in the United Kingdom to both support the existence of a specialist agency and use its services.

The basic philosophy underlying its establishment was that nursing, as a caring profession, should be concerned about the relatively small yet still significant number of its members who find themselves involved in the disciplinary procedures of their regulatory body. Twenty-five years on, that underlying philosophy still holds good. The major change to have occurred is that the potential clientele is now composed of all the nurses, midwives and health visitors on the UKCC's professional register – approximately 630 000 people with current effective registration.

It would be all too easy to castigate the small number of practitioners who have become the subject of complaints alleging misconduct as the delinquents who have brought their profession into disrepute by their reprehensible actions. In some cases that is absolutely true and it is appropriate that those practitioners have their future registration status called into question. To make such judgment in respect of all such practitioners would, however, be to hide from the truth and be tantamount to an abdication of professional responsibility towards colleagues who have cracked under intolerable pressure or are victims of inadequate working environments allowed to exist by those who have now rejected them. The Nurses Welfare Service's explanatory leaflet is appropriately entitled *When the coping becomes too much....*[1] As a disciplinary case, or a case before the committee that considers alleged unfitness to practise due to illness, unfolds it so often becomes all too apparent that the practitioner concerned has been subjected to intolerable levels of stress, either at home, at work, or in both settings simultaneously. Of course there are exceptions, but the majority of nurses, midwives and health visitors are caring, conscientious people with a strong professional commitment. Such practitioners are not immune to the pressures that can sometimes culminate in atypical behaviour.

Origins of the Nurses' Welfare Service

The decade that saw the birth of what became (and is still known as) the Nurses Welfare Service was one which also witnessed a fundamental reappraisal of the whole concept of professional discipline on the part of the one council which helped that organisation into existence and assisted it to establish its important role. Suddenly a subject that had been kept fairly secret was being discussed at conferences, seminars and study days all over the country. This resulted in a significant increase in the level of awareness about the disciplinary aspect of the work of the General Nursing Council (for England and Wales). The Nurses Welfare Service played then, and continues to play, a vital part in the development of a more caring, positive, enlightened philosophy with regard to professional discipline. This philosophy is that rehabilitating an offending practitioner, or one whose inadequate or inappropriate practice has been a result of illness, can be a recognised objective to pursue, while taking the action required to protect the public from unsafe practitioners.

Looking back to 1972, it can be seen that grafting a social work agency that offered support to an individual nurse involved in the disciplinary process on to the statutory body's established process was not an easy task. Extreme caution was necessary to ensure that the service was established on a firm legal base and that it would not interfere in any way with the due process of law by which that body had to investigate and judge complaints against named individuals. It is interesting to look back and note that, in its original terms of reference, the Nurses Welfare Service, through its professional staff, could only become involved in a case after the then Disciplinary Committee had made its decision. Over the next few years the role of the service was the subject of continuous review and evaluation. The result was that the remit of service was steadily extended.

The model on which this service is based is the United Kingdom's statutory Probation and After-Care Service. There are many similarities between the two in that probation officers are social workers operating in a court setting and many of the clients of the Nurses Welfare Service have already been convicted in court and are identified by their connection with the statutory body's disciplinary function. Experience in statutory probation work has therefore proved to be an appropriate background for those who take posts as professional welfare advisers with the Nurses Welfare Service.

The situation now with UKCC, as was the case until 1983 with the General Nursing Council for England and Wales, is that the relationship between the Council and the service is one of sensitivity, delicacy and mutual trust. Some people find it difficult to understand how a statutory body with responsibility for taking disciplinary action against an individual practitioner (in many cases removing their right to practise) can at the same time make possible the offer of a helping hand. Experience has shown that these two concepts are complementary rather than contradictory, provided you accept the basic premise that professional regulation and discipline is about the protection of the vulnerable public and not about punishment. It is also established as essential that the help and support offered must be, and must be perceived to be, separate from the body taking the disciplinary action, even though funded by that body in a majority of cases. This separation is vital from the point of view of potential clients, as it must be abundantly clear to them that they can enter into relationships of trust with the welfare advisers in the certain knowledge that none of the information shared in the course of an interview will be passed on to anyone without prior consent.

Nurses Welfare Trust

To emphasise the separate nature of the service, a trust was established (as a registered charity) at the onset to bear the responsibility for administering the service and raise a substantial part of the money the operation requires. In a large number of cases the UKCC recognises the practitioners' need of support and also recognises that its decision-making will be aided by the kind of background social enquiry reports that, with consent, will be made available by the welfare advisers. In such cases the UKCC formally commissions the work and therefore meets its full cost. The remainder of the income is obtained through voluntary donations and the support of some established charitable trusts. Such income is necessary to meet the costs of providing a service which, by counselling and support at an earlier stage, helps prevent many practitioners deteriorating to that point where report to the statutory body occurs. The number of practitioners who can be assisted is, however, severely limited by the funds available.

The existence of the trust (the Nurses Welfare Trust; registered charity 266994) has given the service professional independence and ensured that its staff are accountable to and able to receive support and advice from the trustees, several of whom are respected practitioners from the social work profession. Separation from the statutory body is therefore seen to be important. So also is the existence of a close working relationship with the statutory body from which the service derives its credibility, much of its stature and its very reason for existence.

Role of the Nurses Welfare Service

The work of the Nurses Welfare Service underwent a dramatic and interesting expansion in 1984 when the UKCC brought into operation its new procedures which allowed it to consider removal from the professional register not only for reasons of 'misconduct', but also where a practitioner's fitness to practise was alleged to be seriously impaired by physical or mental illness. The procedures for considering allegations of misconduct have been explained in Chapter 8 and those for considering possible unfitness to practise due to illness in Chapter 9. Both are the subject of further explanation in Appendix 6. Suffice it here to say that a large number of the practitioners whose fitness to practise is the subject of consideration both need and receive a great deal of specialist support during an extremely difficult and testing time in their lives. One such practitioner, who has been a client of the Service, happily now restored to the register, has very courageously told his story in an article in *Nursing Times*.[2]

The Nurses Welfare Service is, therefore, a specialist social work agency, staffed by qualified professional social workers, which exists to provide casework help and support for any nurse, midwife or health visitor involved in, or at risk of becoming involved in, the disciplinary or fitness to practise procedures of the regulatory system in the United Kingdom. It is an unfortunate fact to have to record, but the volume of preventative work that has been able to be done has always been severely limited by the inadequate funding.

The fundamental premise on which the work is based is that of a voluntary contract between client and welfare adviser. Potential clients of the service may come to its attention by self-referral, referral from other social workers (notably Probation Officers), or referral from concerned professional managers or colleagues. Many who fall in the first category make contact, having been made aware of the existence and role of the service through an introductory leaflet enclosed with the letter sent on behalf of the Preliminary Proceedings Committee to invite a statement in respect of the misconduct alleged. Some others in that category will receive a similar leaflet when invited to attend for medical examinations because concern about their fitness to practise has been expressed. Provided that the individual practitioner gives written consent, the officer of the Nurses Welfare Service involved with the case will be provided with copies of all relevant documents as they are assembled.

The role of the service is not that of appearing at the Professional Conduct Committee or Health Committee as a representative or advocate. That is the task of the officer of the professional organisation or trade union of which the practitioner is a member or of the lawyer the practitioner engages for the purpose. Such a representative is committed to obtaining the best possible outcome of the case for the client. The welfare adviser is concerned with endeavouring to help the client face up to the reality of the situation, even though that may be painful at the time. The files of the Nurses Welfare Service would illustrate the large number of occasions on which it was necessary for its staff to get their clients to face up to the inevitability of removal from the register. Those same files would also illustrate how frequently the individual's acceptance of that fact marked the beginning of their rehabilitation.

There are those who, either for effect or because they are concerned that it might mislead, express concern that the word 'welfare', included in the service's title when it was first created in 1972, still remains there. It does so because the service is concerned with the welfare of individuals, both short-term and long-term. It provides a case-work/counselling service for its clients, enabling them to identify the underlying factors which have brought them to their statutory body's attention. It assists clients to formulate realistic plans to work through the identified problems. It ensures that practitioners are accompanied and supported on what are among the most important yet most lonely days of their lives. It is still there to assist the practitioner when a committee of his or her peers has decided that the public interest requires that they should not be allowed to practise in their chosen profession. Surely all these are aspects of welfare, using that word in its broadest and most constructive sense.

The work of the Nurses Welfare Service

Some of the work of the welfare advisers is undertaken by visiting clients in their homes. Such visits tend to be particularly productive for both adviser and client. The latter normally feels more relaxed and able to talk more freely in the familiarity and security of his or her own home. The fact that the welfare adviser has probably travelled a long way for that home visit tends to be seen as demonstrating his caring attitude. The practitioner – often dismissed from employment and now at risk of losing his or her registration status – is helped by this single gesture to feel valued again. The professional staff of the Service would, were the resources available for their work greater, undertake 'home visits' more frequently, always assuming it was considered appropriate by the adviser and was acceptable to the client.

The work is rarely easy. Indeed, it has become very clear from an early stage of the existence of the Service that (for the welfare adviser) working with a client group composed of fellow professionals in what must still be regarded as a pioneering field of social work demands very special skills. Numerous nurses, midwives and health visitors have difficulty accepting that they need help. This may be because they lack insight into their particular problem – something commonly encountered where it is alcohol- or drug-related. It may be because accepting that you have a need of help tends to be seen by many practitioners as a sign of weakness or an admission of defeat. Added to that, for all of us in the caring professions, is the fact that to be receiving care is a reversal of roles.

One major focus of the work – now, as in the formative years of the service – is that of short-term crisis intervention during the period that clients are actually going through the professional conduct or fitness to practise systems. Anxiety is at least partially allayed. The complexities of the system are explained. The myths and fantasies some practitioners still have about the powers of the Council – for example, that it could send the person to prison or fine them large sums of money – are replaced by the facts.

In addition to such short-term work, each welfare adviser carries a nucleus of long-term cases. For the most part this is made up of practitioners whose names have been removed from the register by one of the two committees empowered to make this decision and who have chosen to maintain contact with the service for the advice and assistance it can give them as they seek to equip themselves for restoration to the register. This aspect of the work can be difficult and frustrating, but in the end often proves extremely rewarding. Convincing a client of the futility of applying for restoration within days of receiving the letter confirming removal from the register is a common experience for all the welfare advisers. By making a premature restoration application a client risks further rejection by his or her profession. For some, however, that further phase of rejection is necessary before they face up to the facts and start to rebuild their lives, either within their chosen profession or in some other area of work.

Social background reports

Reference has already been made to the preparation of social background reports to be presented to the committee considering the case of a practitioner who has voluntarily chosen to accept the assistance of the service. The purpose of preparing such a report is to enable the committee to see the matters which have brought the practitioner to their attention in the context of that individual's personal and professional life. On occasions a social background report reveals a catalogue of disasters of such magnitude that one is left wondering how the practitioner in question managed to keep going so well for so long. A report can also serve to indicate that the incident which has placed the practitioner's registration in jeopardy is the result of momentary aberration when under pressure and needs to be seen in the context of 20 years unblemished, committed, high quality professional service.

The assistance the members of the committees derive from these reports in the difficult decisions they have to make is enormous. Each report is a comprehensive, objective, honest appraisal of the client and his or her circumstances, prepared by someone who is knowledgeable about the committee's role and powers and mindful of its prime responsibility to protect the vulnerable public.

Case histories

Two case histories are provided to illustrate the nature of the work of this important service. Further illustrative material can be found in the 1987/1989 *Report of the Nurses Welfare Trust* and the more recent annual reports of the Nurses' Welfare Service.[3,4,5]

Case history 'A'

Susan, a 34-year-old registered general nurse, with an impeccable professional record, was employed as a sister in an accident and emergency unit at a small general hospital in a quiet provincial town. She had been in post for some 5 years and enjoyed an excellent reputation amongst her professional colleagues as a highly competent sister.

Following the break-up of her marriage, she became acutely depressed and turned to alcohol in an attempt to escape from the unhappy state in which she found herself. Her intake gradually increased to the point where it began to affect her performance at work. Colleagues noticed all was not well but turned a blind eye, making allowances for the difficult time Susan was experiencing in her personal life. Then one day she inadvertently administered the wrong medication to a patient. During the enquiry which followed, a bottle of sherry was discovered in Susan's changing room locker. Her dependency on alcohol had become so acute that she was unable to finish a shift without recourse to the sherry bottle.

She was dismissed from her post and reported to the statutory regulating body for investigation. At this point she made contact with the Nurses' Welfare Service, feeling she was a total failure, having lost her husband, her job and now being faced with the prospect of having her name removed from the professional register. She felt both ashamed and yet relieved that her problem had at last come out into the open. She had become isolated and withdrawn following the failure of her marriage and had experienced a great deal of guilt because of her drinking.

Susan was in need of a lot of support, especially as she did not belong to a staff organisation. The realisation that her professional qualification was at risk convinced her of the need to seek specialist help. She spent eight weeks in a detoxification unit followed by a lengthy course of psychotherapy as an outpatient. The Welfare Adviser remained in close contact, complementing the medical care she was receiving. He also assisted her in the preparation of a statement for consideration by the Preliminary Proceedings Committee which decided that she should be referred to the Health Committee of the UKCC.

With the help of the Nurses Welfare Service, Susan's rehabilitation had begun. She decided to take out an option on a new career in case her name was removed from the register, and was accepted at her local polytechnic on a secretarial/business studies course. Having nursed a large number of people in the local community, she felt so ashamed and embarrassed at meeting them in the street that she dramatically changed her hairstyle in an attempt to lessen the risk of being recognised. She found it difficult to cope with the transition from the caring role of ward sister to the very different skills required for a secretarial course. She needed a lot of encouragement to persevere, especially at times when the old craving for alcohol returned. She joined Alcoholics Anonymous and found this fellowship enormously supportive and helpful in her attempts at maintaining sobriety.

According to the requirements of the Nurses, Midwives and Health Visitors Professional Conduct Rules, she was examined by two independent medical practitioners who prepared reports for the Health Committee of the UKCC. The Welfare Adviser, who by then had been supporting Susan for nearly two years, also prepared a detailed report explaining what had been happening during that time. He concluded that Susan had tackled her problems with courage, determination and realism . . . she had come a long way in restoring her self-respect and pride. She had not had an alcoholic drink for 2 years and had acquired new skills to equip her for alternative employment although at times she had found the going very hard. Finally, it was his view that she had demonstrated, over a 2-year period, that her rehabilitation was successfully accomplished.

Susan attended the Health Committee, which meets in private, accompanied by the Welfare Adviser. She felt very apprehensive but gave a good account of herself. The outcome was favourable and she has recently returned to nursing, a wiser and more mature practitioner after her traumatic experiences of recent years.

Case history 'B'

Sally (aged 38) had not only excelled academically in her RGN training, carrying off most of the prizes, but was regarded by all who had worked with her as an exceptionally conscientious, committed and professional practitioner. She seemed to have an unlimited capacity for work; as well as efficiently running a busy medical ward, she fitted in a demanding Open University course, and on several occasions had to nurse her elderly parents, with whom she lived, through a variety of illnesses. On one such occasion, Sally found herself having to ferry her mother, who was suffering from lymphosarcoma, to and from hospital, and the constant pressure was interfering with her sleep. Rather than approach the notoriously unhelpful staff doctor, she helped herself to eight barbiturate tablets from the ward. By the time this came to light, Sally had commenced midwifery training; she immediately resigned despite the wholehearted support of her managers, fearing that her name would be removed from the register. However, in view of her excellent references, and the many mitigating circumstances, she was allowed to retain her professional qualification.

Sally continued her career with hardly a break, quickly finding a staffing position at another hospital, and was very soon offered a sister's post there. She also began to pursue various management training courses. Again, work pressure was heavy, and her parents' needs and her academic work took up any spare time, on top of which her friends tended to use her, too, as a counsellor and adviser. However, an attempt to lessen the load by working in a quiet local nursing home did not prove satisfactory; she missed the challenge and variety of the hospital setting, and soon applied for a hospital post again. Shortly after this move, pressure began to build up on various fronts.

Firstly, Sally began to suffer various physical ailments, beginning with an acute lumbar disc leading to complications necessitating surgery. She also suffered recurrent mouth ulcers. Her mother, meanwhile, had developed an acute illness culminating in a laparotomy for the removal of a malignant cyst, and Sally spent a lot of time looking after her during her convalescence. Finally, the staffing situation at the hospital had become increasingly parlous, and Sally had constantly to cover for senior hospital staff, and frequently to act up.

When she again developed symptoms in her leg, Sally did not return to her medical advisers, but instead began to take Valium from the ward where she worked. This led to discrepancies in the ward drug register, which were eventually discovered by which time 50 tablets had been misappropriated, over a period of about six months. Sally had used the tablets in a 'sensible' manner, as if they had been prescribed. Her manager stressed that her high standard of work had never altered.

Sally had immediately resigned her post, and was, by the time the Professional Conduct Committee considered her case, working in an antique shop cum art gallery. The Welfare

Adviser who had visited several times had helped her to see clearly how her attempt to be all things to all men was ultimately self-defeating and she understood that, in the end, nothing could justify the theft and self-prescription of drugs. Sally attended the Professional Conduct Committee and it came as no surprise to be told her name was to be removed from the register.

In the aftermath of that decision Sally is in need of, and is receiving, a lot of help from the Nurses Welfare Service in coming to terms with the loss of her professional qualification. She is in a state of bereavement having lost her right to practise in her chosen profession which she had served with distinction for 17 years. She has to live with the stigma of being 'struck off', news of which had spread through her local community by means of a report in the press. Sally also feels an acute sense of failure, having let not only herself down, but also her family, friends and especially her own professional peer group to whom she had previously promised that she would never again abuse the trust placed in her as a nurse. When she reads about the current shortage of nurses she feels guilty that because of her own folly she is no longer allowed to practise. Although she is glad to have a job in the antique shop, she feels uncomfortable and sometimes embarrassed at meeting former patients and colleagues in her new role. Any mention of hospital makes her feel rejected, de-skilled, and useless.

Sally will need a lot of time to work through the pain and hurt which she now feels. She knows that she has the ongoing support of the Service for however long she may need it. Perhaps eventually she may feel ready to apply for the restoration of her name to the professional register.

The messages conveyed by these case histories are reinforced by the verbatim extracts from statements made by former clients of the Nurses Welfare Service quoted in its Annual Reports for 1994/1995 and 1995/1996.[4,5]

Conclusion

The creation and development of the Nurses Welfare Service has been a significant feature of the positive revolution that has been occurring in professional regulation over the last 25 years. Many members of the former General Nursing Council for England and Wales and the present United Kingdom Central Council for Nursing, Midwifery and Health Visiting have said that they would find it very difficult to serve on those committees empowered to remove practitioners' names from the register if the service did not exist. They take support and comfort from the fact that, because realistic and understanding support is available on a continuing basis, their decision to require removal from the register is often the first step towards that individual's rehabilitation. The many nurses, midwives and health visitors who have received support at difficult times in their lives, have become suitably rehabilitated and have since given years of high quality service to their patients and clients, are excellent evidence of the need for and achievements of the Nurses Welfare Service. It is, perhaps, a sad comment with which to close this chapter, but I am not convinced that, if the Nurses Welfare Service did not already exist, a comparable set of pioneers to those who were active in 1972 would succeed in launching it today. That disturbs me greatly, since I contend that a regulatory body disregards an essential aspect of its role if, in the exercise of its disciplinary powers, it acts without thought of remedy or rehabilitation and puts no measures in place to assist persons to regain the ability and authority to practise in their chosen profession, subject always to the overriding public interest.

References

1 *When the coping becomes too much....* Explanatory Leaflet. London: Nurses Welfare Service.
2 Crabtree D. (1990) To Hell and Back. *Nursing Times* **86**, 42.
3 *Nurses Welfare Service – Report of the years 1987 to 1989*. London: Nurses Welfare Service.
4 *Nurses Welfare Service – Annual Report, 1994/1995*. London: Nurses Welfare Service.
5 *Nurses Welfare Service - Annual Report, 1995/1996*. London: Nurses Welfare Service.

Section IV

Views of Professional Regulation

Chapter 11

A View of the Profession: Victims of Change or Agents of Change?

Introduction

My intention in this chapter, by offering a personal view of the profession of which I have now been a part for 42 years, is to challenge those who read it, and particularly the nurses, midwives and health visitors among them, to accept the need to become and remain people who challenge. For convenience, I use the term 'nurses', but intend it to include their fellows in midwifery and health visiting practice.

My contention is that, if they respond to this challenge, they might, as a result, shed the mantle of victims of change which nurses have, I suggest, all too readily borne, and adopt instead that of agents of change. I believe this to be necessary if, in the future, those often anxious, vulnerable and dependent people we call our patients and clients are to receive the services they need and deserve. My further contention is that to continue to opt for the role of victims of change is a betrayal of the interests of those same people.

An uncertain profession

It was my privilege and responsibility to have been a member of the senior professional staff of the profession's regulatory body in my country – the United Kingdom Central Council for Nursing, Midwifery and Health Visiting – during its first 12 years of existence. This provided me with the opportunity to speak at more conferences, seminars and workshops and in more places than I care to remember. Almost without exception, however, that involved me in addressing subjects of someone else's choosing. When I eventually engaged in a retrospective study of the list of subjects I had been asked to address over a period of several years, I found that it was dominated by one particular theme. I realised that the subjects I had been asked to address on a majority of occasions demonstrated the existence (at least in the minds of the organisers of the conferences, seminars and workshops, so possibly also of the participants) of confusion, anxiety, doubt and a great need for reassurance.

Fortunately, even if only in a minority of instances, they also reflected a desire to identify and use the opportunities that have been presenting themselves to break out to a better future for the profession and a better service for the public. Latterly, recognition of the need to put ethical thinking and ethical practice to the fore has been evident, as has something of a search for empowerment. That was a welcome relief. But, taking account of the evidence as a whole, there was more than enough to suggest that the profession was experiencing an identity crisis and was feeling nervous about its current and future role.

The victim phenomenon

Having stated that the challenge to nurses contained in this chapter is to shed the role of victim of the changes promoted by others and, instead, to become an agent of positive change, I must offer some definitions of these contrasted words.

The principal definition of 'victim', found in two major dictionaries with only a modest difference in wording, was 'A living being offered as a sacrifice'. That is not quite the definition I had in mind, though I accept that some of my colleagues in the profession – those who have in recent years been displaced from what had been regarded as key posts through sudden arbitrarily imposed changes that had nothing to do with the care of patients – may think it all too accurate.

What I had in mind was what emerged through the slightly softer definitions, including 'One subjected to suffering or ill-treatment' or 'One who has been hurt by someone or something'.

An 'agent' is clearly something very different. Here my dictionaries provided 'A person who acts or exerts power' and 'A person who has a particular effect which is the means or cause of something happening, for example an "agent of change"'.

The Thesaurus links 'agent' with positive words and phrases, such as 'prime mover' and 'turning point', whereas for 'victim' it offers 'prey' and similar terms. I offer you these definitions in order that you can understand the perspective from which I approach my subject and that we can move forward on the same wavelength.

It is my contention that far too many nurses have, in recent years, become 'prey'. Prey to the whims of others as they have introduced sweeping changes which have often found no justification in the central purposes of health services – that of providing empathetic, competent and effective care for ill and injured people – that of promoting health and preventing disease – that of caring for women during pregnancy, delivery and the post-natal period. But it is also my contention that much of this happened, and was able to happen, because, over many years, practitioners had either not promoted positive and constructive change in and through their practice, or, if they were, had been keeping very quiet about it.

A distorted tradition

This, of course, is a product of one of our profession's distorted traditions. That which, though unwritten, appeared to be saying very powerfully that 'good conduct' meant being compliant and submissive. It is this that has created a scenario in which practitioners, for far too long, pretended that they were coping when they were not, deceived themselves that things were better than they really were, struggled to paper over the cracks and, in the end, let it appear that there was spare capacity in the system when there was not.

Even if you think that something of a caricature – and I hasten to add that I do not – I think that you will recognise that there is a great deal of truth and accuracy in it. Perhaps it has something to do with the 'obedience culture' that gripped the nursing profession from its early days. This was epitomised as long ago as 1874 by Florence Lees, in her publication *A Handbook for Ward Sisters*. In a memorable paragraph she states that the best advice she had ever received in all her career was that from a doctor who told her that, at all times and in all situations, she must respond to his orders immediately and without question![1] I often get the impression that there are still many disciples of Florence Lees at large in the profession in the United Kingdom, busily doing as she says, and thus contributing to the creation and persistence of the 'victim' phenomenon. I suspect that much the same thing can be said of the nursing profession in some other countries.

To have adopted this approach, and still more to continue to adopt this approach, I regard as profoundly unethical. Unethical in respect of those who are currently patients or clients, and still more unethical in respect of those who will be cast in that role in the future, since we need now to think about the services that will be available for them when their need comes. For their sakes, we cannot adopt a 'Sufficient unto the day . . .' approach.

Having described that approach to practice as unethical, I grasp the opportunity to share with you another quotation. Dock, in a paper first published in 1900, states that the earliest advocates of a code of ethics for nurses in America were advised by a physician, 'Be good women, but do not bother with a code of ethics'.[2] Pursuing this point, Johnstone has stated that:

> 'Fortunately, not only have nurses ignored this advice but, since 1973, they have adopted an international code of ethics that recognises and explicates the nurse's independent responsibility and accountability for nursing care'.[3]

She develops this point by her contention that:

> 'Statements that once abrogated the nurse's judgment and personal responsibility and showed dependency on physicians were, in 1973, deleted once and for all from nursing codes of conduct around the world, and thus from nursing philosophy'.

I am pleased to say that, from its first edition in 1983 to its current third (1992) edition, the distorted philosophy to which Johnstone refers has had no place in the UKCC's Code of Professional Conduct with which I have been associated. It finds its origins in the International Council of Nurses Code of Ethics of 1973[4] and has, from the beginning, sought to promote a positive professional revolution, in that it has rejected the 'Good conduct means being compliant and submissive' approach, and replaced it with a declaration that this is no longer the case. This code is, in effect, declaring that 'good conduct' involves being honest, open, questioning and challenging, because these are the qualities, together of course with knowledge and skill, that best serve the interests of patients and clients. There is much evidence to suggest that this UKCC code, together with the several documents that now supplement it, has had a positive impact on the attitudes and activities of many of the practitioners to whom it has been addressed, but there is no room for complacency.

A culture of obedience

The compliant and submissive model of nurse still finds many disciples in the profession, some of them even seeking to support their passive approach to their role by reference to the culture of blind obedience they believe to have been promoted by Florence Nightingale. Johnstone argues, in my view quite correctly, that this is unfair, and has helpfully pointed out, of Nightingale, that, 'Although she had a profound respect for "the rules" and for the "principle of obedience", she was very aware that rules could be restrictive'. She has also emphasised Nightingale's view that nurses required an 'obedience of intelligence, not obedience of slavery'.[5]

There has undoubtedly been progress, but it has not been sufficient to achieve the conversion that I seek. Nurses are still, far too often, treated in a paternalistic and condescending manner. While this is undoubtedly annoying and frustrating, we must surely allow it to stir us into asking ourselves an important and difficult question. Is this situation created entirely by others, or does it result from the fact that we have, as it were, opted into the role of victim and then let others consolidate us in that role?

I suggest that, at least in substantial part, it is a matter of whether opportunities are taken or allowed to pass. Somebody – I cannot now recall who – once said of the French Communist Party that it never missed an opportunity to miss an opportunity. Is it perhaps the case that, in respect of looking to the future, and also in respect of creating a better future with better outcomes for patients and the public at large, the nursing profession in the United Kingdom (and possibly elsewhere) could be characterised by the same words?

Of course, others have played their part. The media, the medical profession and the courts have sometimes been less than helpful, either not understanding or not being willing to accept the role that nurses are capable of filling to the benefit of society. To those sources of obstruction can be added some managers in positions of power in the new National Health Service, striving to apply market principles to a public service, who often seem motivated by thoughts that seem alien to the culture that nurses wish to promote and in which they wish to practise well.

Changing the culture

The time has surely come to break the mould in a comprehensive way. That is to say that, while recognising the role played by others in creating the victim culture, members of the nursing profession, both individually and collectively must recognise that, by their compliance, by the absence of articulate challenge and by their reluctance to be provocative, they have largely chosen the role of victims for themselves.

The time has surely come for each and every practitioner to demonstrate a personal and professional commitment to bring about positive change in nursing practice and in health care more generally. So what is to be done if we are to shed the role of victims of change and adopt that of agents of change?' My response to my own rhetorical question has two parts. First, that we must bring a deeper understanding of ethics to the heart of our practice and use it as a platform for our professional practice and for the explanation of that practice to others. Second, that we must constantly re-examine ourselves, our practice and the context in which we practise, the focus being the identification of the things that need to be included in that practice in order best to meet the needs and serve the interests of patients and clients.

The scope of practice

The latter part of that response leads me to comment briefly about an important document published by the UKCC. I refer to the document entitled *The Scope of Professional Practice*. As a person directly involved in the preparation of this text, at one level I make no great claims for it. Indeed, I have often presented it to audiences as a collection of statements of the obvious. And yet, given what it is seeking to achieve, at another level I make substantial claims about this document and its potential to achieve enormous and positive change in professional practice and the attitudes of practitioners.

In effect, given the fences that had been allowed to be erected around the practice of individuals, given the comfortable ruts into which too many had settled, and given also the limitations which some nurses in management positions had unreasonably imposed on the practice of those who reported to them, this document was fairly revolutionary.

It is revolutionary because it rejects the suggestion that we should think of practice as having limitations or boundaries and concentrates instead on the 'scope' of professional practice. It is of the greatest possible importance, because its key theme and solid intention is that of 'meeting the needs and serving the interests of patients', first stated in paragraph 9 and then restated and embellished frequently thereafter.

To the individual practitioner, irrespective of the post that they hold, through this document the Council is, in effect, saying: '*You* look carefully and critically at yourself. *You* examine critically and in detail your own practice. *You* look at your practice in context, all the while thinking about the requirement that you will meet the needs and serve the interests of your patients. And through this critical self-examination, *you* identify those activities which, if only you could absorb them into your practice, would help to meet that important objective.'

It is also, in effect, saying to practitioners that, having done all of those things, you should ask yourself if you have the knowledge and skill to develop your practice. If 'Yes' is your answer, shouldn't you be declaring your intentions to your line managers? If 'No' is your answer, recognising that your patients would be better served if you did have the knowledge and skill to develop the scope of your practice, shouldn't you be doing something about it and asking your managers to assist to that end? Surely the answer is that you should.

The way to use the document entitled *The Scope of Professional Practice* (the full text of which is reproduced at Appendix 5) is, therefore, to use the freedoms it offers. To use, that is, the freedom and encouragement it offers to focus on the scope of practice and to reject the concept of practice as having boundaries or limitations. To give to each practitioner the freedom to develop their approaches to practice and the support they require to that end. To encourage initiative and innovation, provided that it is properly directed. The barriers, in the United Kingdom, with very few exceptions, are those of custom and practice and not of law.

This is about being an agent of change rather than a victim of change. It is about starting, always, with the question 'What should I be doing to meet the needs and serve the interests of my patients?' and, having identified the answer, proceeding accordingly. It is also about recognising that good quality care is often best provided by a good quality team.

I sincerely hope that the claims I have made for this brief publication prove to be correct, in that we will see health care teams engaging in more truly collaborative working, see evidence of greater flexibility in practice and see an enhanced role for registered nurses, midwives and health visitors. That, however, depends on their ability and willingness to be creative, innovative and bold. But it also depends on the willingness of their managers to enable and facilitate rather than restrict them in their endeavours – on their willingness to see moves into the best and most constructive clinical supervisory role, as distinct from a conventional and often narrow managerial role.

The prize that is there to be grasped is a substantial one. It is one which can offer satisfying practice to the accountable practitioner, while at the same time providing improved care for patients and clients. Surely that combination is worth striving to achieve!

A theme for our times

The lyrics of the songs that Stephen Sondheim has written for his many stage musicals are, for the most part, very profound. In this respect they are quite untypical of this musical genre, and, for this and other reasons, worthy of close attention. Significant and telling comments about the human condition in general and relationships between individuals reward the person who pays careful attention to his words. More significant still is the fact that these lyrics often contain a call to action, and state the consequences of failure to act.

A good example of this is found in the wonderful (though very difficult to sing) song *Everybody says don't* from Sondheim's intriguingly titled musical play *Anyone Can Whistle*. The repeated advice to be cautious, to hold back, to avoid taking action that might be construed by others as challenging, is stridently rejected by a clarion call to action. I extract from this song the message that if you do not try, you have already failed. I suggest that there is a theme for our times in that lyric. I hope that the message it conveys is both noted and acted upon by members of the nursing profession.

Changing the culture

Many readers may conclude that, in this personal view of the state of my profession in 1997, I have painted an excessively bleak picture. On reflection I suspect that this may be true. I readily concede that some marvellous and innovative developments in nursing practice, initiated by thoughtful, committed and brilliant practitioners are there to be observed. I am pleased that many of them reach the pages of the professional journals. It would, however, be just as foolish to become euphoric and conclude that they represent the current norm in nursing practice as it would to become excessively gloomy and regard the norm as that represented by the respondents in the Professional Conduct Committee case studies set out in Chapter 13. What matters is that the bulk of the profession move in the direction of the former rather than the latter, and do it soon.

Fortunately the infrastructure is in place to help make such positive developments possible. There is scope in British law for major development in nursing practice, the purpose of which is not to inflate the image of the practitioner but to better meet the needs and serve the interests of patients. The profession's regulatory body has stated its expectations of its practitioners in clear terms, and is encouraging an innovative approach to professional practice.

Individual nurses and their regulatory body are in this together. The overriding purpose of the statutory regulation of nursing (that this book has been describing) is that of service to the public and protection of the public. In order to honour this laudable intention it is necessary for the nursing profession to use all the methods at its disposal and within its authority to make available to the public nursing care that is competent, accessible, effective and appropriate. This can only be achieved if (a) the organisation that bears the responsibility for regulation of the profession is alert and innovative in the fulfilment of its role, and (b) individual nurses adopt a dynamic approach to their role, accept the responsibility for continuing critical reappraisal of their practice as health care changes and strive to achieve their full potential in the service of the public.

References

1 Lees F. (Quoted in *History of the General Nursing Council for England and Wales, 1919–1969*. Bendall E. & Raybould E.)
2 Dock L.L. (1900) in *Short papers on nursing subjects*. New York: M. Louise Longerway.
3 Johnstone M-J. *Bioethics: A nursing perspective*, Second Edition (1994). Marrickville/ London: Harcourt Brace & Co.
4 *Code for Nurses* (1973). Geneva: International Council of Nurses.
5 Nightingale F. (Quoted in *Bioethics: A nursing perspective*, Second Edition (1994), by M-J. Johnstone. Manickville/London: Harcourt Brace & Co.)

Chapter 12

How Does it Look from the Outside?

In a short letter published in *The Independent* on 24 February 1996, Mr Leo Haynes challenged the recently expressed opinion of the then President of The Law Society that the role of a professional regulatory body was to identify and then serve the interests of the members of the profession. I am indebted to him for the crisply stated reminder that this is not the case, and that their primary reason for existence is to serve the interests of the public at large.

I am indebted to Mr Leo Haynes for that, and for providing, in such a few words, a comprehensive reminder for all regulatory bodies about the role that they are intended to fulfil.

I read that salutary reminder just a few months after retiring from the staff of the UKCC which I had served since its establishment in 1983, having also been directly involved in the regulation of my profession through the largest of the replaced regulatory bodies for a number of years before that date. In the period since retirement from my previous salaried employment I have continued my professional activities through conference papers, lectures and seminars presented for nurses, midwives and health visitors, and thus have maintained links with many people in current practice. In addition I have been able to increase significantly the amount of time committed to my voluntary role as the Chairman of a Community Health Council, one of its duties being to conduct monitoring visits of hospitals and other health care facilities.

It can therefore be seen that, while I have not shed my professional hat, I have found the time to wear my consumer hat more often and become more involved and active in the consumer activist role. My activities in the first category provide me with an opportunity to talk not only to the students but also to those who teach them. Meanwhile, as the Chairman of my Community Health Council, participating more often than was previously possible in monitoring visits to a wide range of clinical facilities in my own area, I meet not only students on clinical placements, but also the registered nurses, midwives and health visitors in those same settings. This combination of experiences has proved most enlightening.

The case for greater openness

That enlightenment has brought me to the conclusion that the professional regulatory bodies generally, and not least that for my own profession, must do much more not only to communicate to the world what their role is, but openly to demonstrate that their public interest responsibilities are being comprehensively honoured. I make this statement from my position as a continued and passionate believer in the importance of professional self-regulation. Were that not my position I would not, for example, have voluntarily given my time to promote that cause in Romania as one of my post-retirement projects.

I repeat here my earlier declaration that, for me, one of the hallmarks of any occupational group seeking to espouse the title 'profession' is that it is willing and able to accept the responsibility of regulating itself, not in the profession's interests, but those of the public which it exists to serve. To that I must add, passionate believer in professional self-regulation that I am, that I believe it will only survive, and will only deserve to survive, if it is seen to achieve its stated purpose. Failure to achieve this, particularly if that smacks in any way of professional self-interest, will lead to its destruction. Mark this well, for it is central to the concerns and proposals that I lay before you later in this chapter. It might also be wise to remind yourself of the essential elements and core principles of professional regulation described in Chapter 2. These core principles should, I contend, be found at the heart of the regulatory system, and all of the elements described must be in place and properly operative if it is to be comprehensive and effective. So then, to respect my chapter heading, how does it look from the outside, or at least from my unusual, if not unique version of the outside?

The first thing that I notice from the outside is that, speaking first of my own profession, so very little is heard of its regulatory body, of that body's role and of the ways in which it is performing its role. And I say that as a person with effective registration with the Council so receiving any items it mails to practitioners, as a person on the mailing list who receives all Council circulars and other documents it issues, as a regular reader of the professional journals and as a person active with my Community Health Council and serving on the National Standing Committee of the Association of Community Health Councils, so seeing anything that reaches those organisations from the regulatory bodies for the health professions. I confess that I had not realised how uninformed about the work of my own professional regulatory body, and the regulatory bodies for other health professions to which it relates, I would be once separated from their daily activity. I would suggest that, if this is true of me and my profession, it is likely to be just as true for others.

The message of this is, surely, that it is not sufficient simply to do what is required. If you profess to serve the public interest you must let it be known what you are doing. Only in that way can judgment be passed on you. Only in that way can it be seen that your accountability to the public is being honoured. Only in that way can it be seen that you have any relevance at all. I find it interesting, and somewhat ironic to note that, while the British Medical Association, the Royal College of Nursing and other membership organisations whose primary, though not only role, is to represent the interests of their members within the professions, get a great deal of attention in the press, those whose primary responsibility is to serve the public interest through the regulatory process get very little.

If the only occasions on which the professional regulatory bodies come to the attention of the public through the press are those on which it is suggested that they have not faced up to their regulatory responsibilities in an appropriate manner and with appropriate weight, it cannot be surprising if the public and politicians then react in a hostile manner.

The case for critical self-appraisal

That leads me to the conclusion that the regulatory bodies must take a critical look at themselves and consider, each of them, how they should remedy this deficit. If they are doing something in the public interest, they should be letting it be known what they are doing. And if, on such critical self-examination, they cannot find any good public interest news to share, they should surely be asking why they are content to take such a minimalist view of their role.

Earlier in this chapter I indicated that, if the only occasions on which a regulatory body comes to the attention of the public through the press is when there is concern about a decision it has made, that body should not be surprised if it is challenged and its role called into question. This leads me on to say, again in respect of my own profession, though expressing a concern that I believe is transferable, that some decisions made by the relevant committees appear perverse in the extreme and impossible to understand. When I was directly involved, managing that part of the UKCC's work concerned with considering allegations of misconduct, I accept that surprising decisions were made from time to time. Unless they were particularly perverse (and on rare occasions they were), I could manage to explain them if asked by practitioners I met, or the press, or others. The operative phrase there is 'if asked by the press'. More often than not the press did not ask, choosing to report only what they saw on the surface – for example, that the nurse who had neglected a patient had not been removed from the register.

I believe that this problem or difficulty is so severe, and so important, that it cannot be neglected. I also believe that, if neglected, it might contribute to the downfall of the professional regulatory systems. That, I believe, must be avoided, for it would be contrary to the public interest. So I have some firm proposals to make.

My first proposal is that, on each and every occasion when the professional conduct committee for my own profession, or the equivalent committee of any other professional regulatory body, having established that the facts alleged are proved to the required high standard, and having decided that those facts amount to misconduct in a professional sense, decides *not* to remove a practitioner from the register, it should be required to determine and state its reasons for that decision. My further proposal is that, on each occasion when such a committee decides to *restore* to the register a person who had previously been removed for misconduct, it should be required to determine and state its reasons. I suspect that the very fact of having to do that would have an impact on the decision on many occasions. I believe that such a practice would help to restore and maintain confidence in the regulatory systems.

I suggest that the bodies would have little to fear from such a practice on those occasions where, for example, the person who had not been removed was a victim of the environment in which they had worked, the deficits in which she or he had drawn to the attention of those concerned, but had then been left to carry on against the odds. I also suggest, in respect of restoration applications, that there would be little to fear where convincing evidence of genuine remorse and true rehabilitation had emerged.

My second proposal is that the same requirement to state reasons be imposed on the Preliminary Proceedings Committees when deciding to issue a formal caution to a practitioner, but not refer the case for hearing with a view to removal. There is a concern that decisions of this kind might be made inappropriately and thus prove contrary to the public interest. The action I propose would resolve that anxiety.

The case for vigilance

My recent experience has led me to feel concerned about the possibly excessive trust which the regulatory bodies appear to show in those other organisations or institutions involved in the process of education and training which renders students eligible for registration. Once again I speak primarily of the profession which I know best because I am part of it, but once again I suspect that at least some of my concern is transferable.

Wearing my consumer hat, I now find myself visiting clinical facilities in which students, supernumerary in status, are placed as a required part of their pre-registration education and training. All too often they seem to be isolated and a bit lost, with insufficient contact, assistance and oversight from their teachers, and not able to get sufficient quality time from the limited number of registered nurses in the setting in which they are placed. This is not how it is meant to be, but it is often how it is. And it generates cynicism and dissatisfaction in all concerned. I have to ask if this is a satisfactory way of preparing our future practitioners.

This suggests to me that there sometimes seems to be far too great a gap between the regulatory bodies and the organisations and institutions directly involved in the business of preparing people to be admitted to their professional registers. Far too great a gap, that is to say, between those who are determining the policies and those meant to deliver something that matches those policies. I detect a great deal of cynicism developing around this point.

In some cases it might be the result of faults in the legislation, in which case they should be exposed and challenged. In some other cases it might be a question of the resources available to exercise the oversight, in which case that should be exposed. Perhaps in some others, it is simply a matter of inertia on the part of certain individuals. If that register – that public interest register – is to mean anything, admission to it ought to mean something very significant indeed. The resultant practitioners ought to have not only the appropriate knowledge and skill, but also the appropriate understanding and attitudes. Does the system achieve that? Does the regulatory body know whether it achieves that? I simply record my concern and pose these questions.

The case for advice and guidance

In both Chapters 2 and 6 I have argued that, if a regulatory body possesses the awesome power to remove a person from the register and prevent them from practising in their chosen profession, it is essential that it provide practitioners with documented advice which indicates, in general terms, what it expects of them. This published information can then also be used to help inform the public what they may expect from members of that profession and provide for them a yardstick for measuring the performance of practitioners they encounter. Slowly and steadily, such statements (for example the UKCC's Code of Professional Conduct, and the General Medical Council's document *The Duties of a Doctor*) infiltrate the minds of persons in Government Departments and begin to be quoted in documents emerging from the Department of Health and the NHS Executive. In this way they have the additional merit of exerting an influence on policy.

It therefore concerns me greatly that there are some regulatory bodies which have not yet recognised the importance of preparing and publishing some form of document which states, to the practitioners themselves but also to the wider public, their expectations of those registered practitioners. I believe that they owe it to their practitioners to do so. Still more to the point, I believe that they owe it to the public that they do so.

The case for competence

I turn now to the important issue of competence or incompetence. When I was managing that part of the UKCC's work that was concerned with investigating and hearing allegations of misconduct, it was a matter of concern to me that the relevant committee could only regard serious incompetence as a matter of misconduct threatening an individual's registration if that incompetence could be proved to be wilful and/or reckless. While I believe that the belated coming to my profession of a system of three-yearly periodic registration is an advance, and that, in order to be able to renew registration, a person must now produce evidence of at least 5 days of relevant study during the previous three-year registration period, we deceive and delude ourselves if we think that this miraculously deals with the competence and incompetence issue.

The UKCC has a splendid provision in primary legislation to allow it to address this matter. I refer to the very same words in section 12 of the Nurses, Midwives and Health Visitors Act 1979 which have provided the power to establish the Health Committee and its associated procedures, now in its nineteenth year of operation. The Council has the power to make rules determining 'the circumstances in which, and the means by which a person may, for misconduct or otherwise, be removed from the register'.[1] The entire Health Committee procedures, described in detail in Chapter 9, have been developed from those two words 'or otherwise'.

It is surely appropriate, therefore, to pose a supplementary question. If that source of power can be used so effectively to protect the public from persons whose fitness to practise is seriously impaired by illness, should it not also be used to develop procedures to deal, in the public interest, with those practitioners who, in spite of all efforts to improve them, are intractably incompetent and thus a danger to the public? I suggest that the UKCC should take steps to equip itself with a system to achieve such public protection without delay, and not wait to see if the new periodic registration requirements make everyone perpetually competent. I accept that it was absolutely right to put in place some requirements to apply when registration is renewed that make that important step involve something more significant than simply paying a fee. But I also believe that the means should be put in place to deal with the practitioner who, in spite of all the efforts to overcome the problem, remains intractably incompetent. Failure to introduce such measures when primary legislation makes it possible might be construed as neglecting the public interest.

In this context I place on record the fact that, while I am pleased that the General Medical Council (GMC) has introduced its new performance procedures through new legislation, I have two serious concerns as a result. One is that the system might be exposed to possible abuse, by using it to steer into a private forum matters that the public would regard as possible misconduct and that ought to be addressed in a public hearing. The second is that it carries the risk of creating the delusion that all medical practitioners who do not come to the attention of the GMC's new procedures are thereby competent.

Just as I think that my own profession's regulatory body should use the opportunity provided for it by primary legislation to develop procedures to deal with the incompetent practitioner, so I also think that the GMC should introduce a requirement that its practitioners do more than just pay money to renew their registration. Apply this, if you will, to all other professions which exist to serve the public. Surely if you are really concerned about the vulnerable public, the incompetent practitioner must be just as much in your sights as the 'bad' practitioner or the 'unfit to practise due to illness' practitioner?

Openness revisited

I turn to the subject of public access to the deliberations of the full regulatory body and of its various committees which debate matters and determine policies, all of which are intended to be related to their public interest role. It now seems to me to be essential that, other than when dealing with private personnel or health matters, all such meetings should be accessible to the public. I believe that there is nothing to fear from this, but simply strength to be gained. I now find it odd that, while the Community Health Council which I chair, with its responsibility of representing the interests of its public to the NHS, is required by law to conduct its affairs in public, this is not the case with the regulatory bodies. So how does it look from the outside? Too secretive, is the conclusion I must reach.

A danger perceived

In bringing this important chapter to a close, there is one final concern that I must share with you. Rightly or wrongly, I sense that, the more the United Kingdom Government, in common with governments in some other countries, pursues its deregulation policy in various aspects of life, the greater is the temptation for existing statutorily established regulatory bodies to opt for a minimalist approach to their roles and responsibilities and to be reluctant to rock the boat for fear of being threatened by Government. This, I contend, is a wrong approach to take. Taking the health care scene as an example, it would be hypocritical of, for example, the UKCC or the GMC to state, through their published documents, their expectations of practitioners, but to care not at all that the settings in which those practitioners have to match those aspirations obstruct them in their endeavours.

The work of any regulatory body to protect the public cannot ever be performed effectively if that body is neglecting the context of practice. It can never be right for a regulatory body to tell its practitioners that they must not be compliant and submissive in the face of things that pose risks, but then itself be compliant and submissive.

Conclusion

So, once again, how does it look from the outside? It looks, I have to say, as if the regulatory bodies are not making their presence adequately felt in the cut and thrust world in which health care is now delivered, and that, I believe, smacks of betrayal of both practitioners and the public. If it is the case that there is fear of what a Government, out of its enthusiasm for deregulation, might do to the regulatory bodies, I contend that the best thing to do is to demonstrate to the public the importance of what you do in their interests and how you do it, and get them on your side. This requires an openness which, perhaps, has not been a traditional feature of regulatory bodies. That Biblical quotation which states (depending on the translation you turn to) 'By their deeds (or fruits) you shall know them' would appear to be relevant here. Surely a quotation worth considering in examining the performance of any regulatory body.

In the course of a conference paper presented in 1994 to an audience drawn from many professions I stated this:

> 'If any one of us does it badly – or appears to be self-serving and professionally precious or protective – or fails to use positively and constructively the legislation that we have – or fails to identify the deficiencies in that legislation and seek remedies – or fails to operate a system which is manifestly fair, efficient and accessible – we let down every professional regulatory body and endanger the principle of self-regulation. In doing so we also let down those other occupational groups who aspire to regulatory status: . . . the essential components of professional regulation in our times must include constant reappraisal and constant striving for improvement.'[2]

Although now viewing the subject from a slightly altered perspective, I still adhere without reservation to that statement. We must keep that in mind. And we must *always* remember that this cachet of professional regulation is not for adornment – it is for application.

References

1 *Nurses, Midwives and Health Visitors Act 1979*, section 12. London: HMSO.
2 Pyne R. (1996) *The Case for Professional Regulation* (unpublished seminar paper). London: Walker Martineau, Solicitors.

Section V
Case Studies

The reader who has read the book to this point and considered carefully the information, explanation and arguments set out in Sections I to IV inclusive, should now have a reasonable understanding of professional regulation and the manner in which the nursing, midwifery and health visiting professions are currently regulated in the United Kingdom. The reader should also be aware of what the author regards as the essential elements of regulation and have noted that the International Council of Nurses has enunciated an important set of 12 principles as the foundation for any professional regulatory process.

This section is different in character. Against the background of what has gone before, it invites the reader to consider, either alone or in partnership with others, a selection of case studies.

Those in Chapter 13 ask the reader to regard herself or himself as a member of the Professional Conduct Committee (see particularly Chapter 8) and apply the legal processes and procedures described. Chapter 14 is different again, since it presents examples of the kind of dilemmas sometimes faced by individual members of the profession as they strive to be the kind of practitioners their regulatory body wishes them to be, but often in less than ideal circumstances.

The purpose of this section is, therefore, to demonstrate some aspects of professional regulation in operation and to provide discussion and study material to aid professional development and understanding of this important subject.

Chapter 13

Professional Conduct Committee Case Studies: 'Could This Happen Where You Work?'

(To be considered in association with Chapters 5 to 9 inclusive)

For the individual or group now wishing to go further into this aspect of regulation and to stimulate discussion, a number of case studies are set out in this chapter.

The case studies are based directly on actual cases considered by the Professional Conduct Committee since 1994. They are in précis form, since each of them reduces to a few paragraphs of text what emerged before the Committee over several hours or even days. They ask you to adopt the role of a member of the Professional Conduct Committee and to decide what decision you would have made, faced with the evidence described. The heading of this chapter is deliberate, since the all too frequent assumption is that the kind of incidents or practices described only happen to other people and in their work settings. Since the events described really happened, it is wise to note them and to ask yourself 'Could this happen where I work?', and if the answer is even as modest as 'Possibly', to take preventative measures without delay.

The decisions made by the Committee in these cases, together with some supplementary comments, are provided in Appendix 1. I suggest that reference be made to that section only after each case has been read, considered and discussed.

Case A1: Owner/manager of registered nursing home

The respondent in this case was a registered nurse and midwife of 30 years experience, who had additional qualifications in health education, family planning and counselling. She was a social science graduate.

She was the subject of 13 charges. These included allegations that she adopted the practice of leaving patients tied to commode chairs with wide crepe bandages, of slapping and verbally abusing patients, of leaving the home on one occasion with no registered nurse on duty, of catheterising patients and administering enemas to patients routinely and unnecessarily, of having adopted without justification the practice of feeding patients food in liquidised form, of a failure in the administration of medicines and of disconnecting the night call bell on a number of occasions.

At the time that the home was purchased by the respondent several years earlier it was registered for 12 residents in the medical, post-operative and elderly care categories. After extension it was registered for 19 residents, the categories being unchanged. The property took the form of a large detached house on three floors. The respondent was both the registered owner and the designated person in charge.

There were four witnesses called to support the charges. The first was the manager of the Registration and Inspection Unit of the Health Authority with which the nursing home was registered. She described how, following a number of complaints to the Health Authority, she made an unannounced visit of inspection on a weekday afternoon and found the home staffed by two care assistants only. Information gleaned on this occasion led to an investigation involving interviews with a number of potential witnesses. This in turn led to the closure of the home by the Health Authority and the charges which the respondent now faced before the Professional Conduct Committee. The second and third witnesses were women who had been employed at the nursing home in the capacity of care assistants. Both had considerable experience in care of the elderly in hospitals and other nursing homes, so had something against which to measure what they described as having occurred. The final witness was a registered nurse who had worked as an agency nurse at the home for one shift only and was disturbed by the practices she observed and described.

In response to the charges, the lawyer representing the respondent called her in evidence. There were nine other defence witnesses. Two of these had been employed for periods as care assistants, 1 as a cook, one as a general assistant not involved in care. The others were a retired hospital social worker who had formerly directed people to this home, a regular visitor from a local church and relatives of former residents. The respondent denied all the charges. The care assistant witnesses accepted that some restraint by bandaging was used, but described it differently and saw it as justifiable. Their position in respect of liquidised food was again to argue that it was justified in the circumstances.

The respondent's lawyer challenged the credibility of the prosecution witnesses and alleged a vendetta against the respondent. He also drew particular attention to the Health Authority's willingness to register the home for an increased number of residents 3 years earlier and its apparent relative satisfaction with what it had seen in an announced visit just 6 weeks before it received the anonymous complaints which precipitated another visit leading to this case.

After hearing evidence for more than 2 days and as a result of long deliberation, the committee found proved two charges of tying residents to commodes, two of slapping residents and one of verbal abuse of a resident and that of leaving the home without a registered nurse on duty. It also found proved the charges that the unnecessary liquidisation of food and administration of enemas had become routine practices.

In the next stage of the hearing the respondent denied that the proven charges were misconduct in a professional sense when considered in context.

What is your view of this, taking account of the Code of Professional Conduct and other advice distributed by the UKCC? Which of these proven charges do you regard as misconduct?

If you decide that any of them are misconduct what decision would you then make about this respondent's registration status? Will you take no action, leave her on the register and possessed of the right to practise, or remove her from the register?

Case A2: Senior nurse manager and night sister of a medium security forensic unit for clients with learning disabilities

Respondent A in this case (the senior nurse manager) was a registered nurse for the mentally handicapped and registered general nurse of more than 20 years standing, the majority of his practice being based upon the former qualification. At the time of the incidents leading to the charges he had been the senior nurse manager of the secure unit for 8 years.

Respondent B (the night sister) was a registered nurse for the mentally handicapped and had held a post as night sister in the medium security unit for 8 years at the time of the incidents leading to the charges.

Respondent A was the subject of nine charges. These were to the effect that (1) he had prevented a resident client (X) from leaving the unit when he had no power to do so, (2) that he attempted to seclude X without proper reason, (3) that he allowed and encouraged other resident clients to remove the clothes of X, (4) that he allowed and encouraged other resident clients to restrain X, (5) that he spoke in an inappropriate manner to X, (6) that he struck X on the back of his head, (7) that he ordered a more junior member of staff to complete a 'Violent Incident Form' providing incomplete and false information and then countersigned it, (8) that he completed a 'Use of Seclusion Form' by inserting false information, and (9) that he omitted to tell the on-call doctor called in to see X that it had been necessary to employ mouth-to-mouth resuscitation and administer oxygen following his collapse.

Respondent B was the subject of three charges. These were to the effect (1) that, although the night sister in charge of the unit at the time, she failed to inquire why oxygen was needed for administration to X, (2) that she failed to complete or properly complete the various records that were required, and (3) that she failed to report in adequate terms an incident involving X which had occurred during the period in which she was in charge of the unit.

Despite all efforts to secure their attendance and substantial delay as a consequence, neither respondent attended the hearing.

The essential circumstances of the case, as they emerged from the evidence given by six witnesses, were that, shortly before the hand-over from day to night staff on the unit, there was a minor fracas between X and another resident client. Members of the day staff dealt with the situation, separated the parties and talked to them individually. X was sitting watching television at 8 PM when respondent A entered the unit, together with respondent B who was arriving for duty. They were told of the incident. Respondent A immediately ordered that X, but not the other client involved, must be taken to his room and sent to bed. Two members of staff took action to enforce this instruction and, not surprisingly, found the client resentful. Once in his room he became aggressive and struck out at one of the members of staff. That staff member (a staff nurse) sought assistance, and respondent B arrived but quickly left again.

Respondent A then arrived in the client's room. X told him he was unhappy and intended to leave the unit which, given the terms of his residence, was within his rights. He was not aggressive at this stage. He was told by respondent A that he could not leave. Respondent A then instructed the staff nurse to assist him take X to the seclusion room. Once in the seclusion room X was told by respondent A to remove his clothes. He refused, so respondent A called three other resident clients and told them to undress him. This they did, X resisting as vigorously as his own physical limitations allowed. In doing so he lashed out and a blow struck respondent A who then told the other clients to restrain him. They brought him to the ground, by then clad only in underpants, and sat on him. By now there was blood on the floor, and X was observed to have a cut on his forehead. One witness stated that respondent A hit the client on the head, stating 'You hit me, you bastard, now I'm hitting you'.

At this stage X suddenly collapsed and, it was said, ceased breathing. The staff nurse attempted some external cardiac massage, while respondent A gave mouth-to-mouth resuscitation. Respondent B brought an oxygen trolley, and oxygen was administered by respondent A. X recovered and was taken to his room in what was described as a dazed and confused state. A doctor was subsequently called to see him, but he was not told of the collapse or the resuscitative treatment provided.

Respondent A dictated to the staff nurse what he should write on the 'Violent Incident Form' and himself inaccurately completed a 'Use of Seclusion Form'. Respondent B , who was in charge of the ward for that night, neither reported the incident in the various ways it should have been reported, ascertained why the oxygen trolley had been required, or adequately addressed the matter in her hand-over the following morning.

The matters came to light because the day staff nurse who had been involved from the outset (and who had remonstrated when the manager involved other resident clients) reported the facts to more senior managers, thus precipitating an urgent investigation.

X, who was the subject of this treatment, was described to the committee as 'a young 21-year-old with a borderline learning disability'. He also had a left-sided hemiplegia which made for 'an ungainly gait and ... his left arm was not a lot of use'. He was said to be 'not prone to aggression'. He was residing in the unit as a condition of a bail order, but was not detained under any section of the Mental Health Act.

In her evidence the Executive Director of the relevant NHS Trust who had been responsible for the conduct of the local disciplinary hearings in respect of these respondents told the committee that, in the course of that hearing, respondent A had admitted most of the alleged facts, but did not admit that he had actually administered oxygen to X or that X had stopped breathing. In respect of respondent B, the witness said that respondent B said she had not questioned respondent A about the details of the incident or why he had wanted the oxygen because he was her superior. This was apparently her standard response to the questions asked of her. Her explanation for the inadequate report at hand-over was that she had no direct knowledge of the incident, that she had not asked her superior about it, so she passed on only that which she knew.

The standard of proof required in law by the Committee is that the members must be satisfied so that they are sure. Against this necessarily hard standard, they found the facts alleged against respondent A in charges 1, 3, 4, 7, 8 and 9 proved. The Committee also found the facts alleged against respondent B in all three charges proved.

Before considering its decision in the case, the Committee received further information about each respondent's employment record. This made it clear that respondent A had every reason to be aware of the unit's policies and procedures concerning seclusion and violent incidents, since he had written them. It was also apparent that he had taken many opportunities to attend both internal and external training events about a wide range of matters relevant to his area of practice. In respect of respondent B, the Executive Director stated that she had attended a limited number of internal events, but added the surprising words 'There is no evidence of her attending any external training events, but that is not particularly surprising given that she is a Night Sister'.

What is your view of this case, taking account of the UKCC's expectations of people on its register? Noting the charges which were proved by the evidence, would you have regarded these as misconduct in a professional sense? If so, what decision will you then make about each respondent's registration status? Neither had been the subject of previous complaint to the Council or their employer. Will you take no action,thus leaving them on the register, or administer a formal caution, or remove their names from the register? It does not have to be the same decision for each, since their involvement was not the same.

Case A3: Registered midwife in independent practice

The respondent in this case was a midwife in independent practice. She worked in partnership with two other midwives. She chose not to attend the hearing before the Professional Conduct Committee. The charge which this respondent faced was to the effect that, whilst practising as a midwife in independent practice with the partnership, she failed to properly manage the antenatal care and early labour of a client and that, in consequence she was guilty of misconduct in a professional sense. There was no admission of the charge. Evidence was given by the respondent midwife's client and six other witnesses.

The circumstances of the case were unusual, in that the client concerned had been receiving antenatal care from the hospital and community midwives of an NHS Trust until the 37th week of her pregnancy. It was her wish that her baby be born at home, but she was advised against that because, at the 37-week stage, the baby was in a breech position. Faced with this situation, she consulted an obstetrician who succeeded in performing an external cephalic version. It was then arranged through the obstetrician that a further scan be performed 6 days later. The conclusion of the specialist ultra-sonographer performing that scan was that the baby was small against dates and that further scans were advisable. It was at this stage that the client made contact with the independent midwifery practice.

The evidence indicated that the client discussed the need for further scans with the respondent midwife and was told by her that she did not feel that they were necessary. The respondent saw and examined the client again on her due date and one of her partners did so 7 days and 14 days later. On the latter occasion, the client now being 14 days post-term, arrangements were made for her to have some CTG monitoring at a private hospital unit 2 days later. This monitoring was performed by a midwife at the hospital. This midwife was not clinically involved in the case, but performed the monitoring as an agent for the independent practice and handed the trace record to the client to give to the respondent.

Two days later the client again attended the specialist ultrasonographer for a further scan. He was concerned at that stage because, although there was evidence of physical growth since the previous scan, he believed the baby to be still small for date and detected a reduction in the fluid around the baby and a reduction in placental blood flow. He accepted, however, that the general movement of the baby and his more subtle observations suggested that, at that stage, the baby was satisfactory. He was sufficiently concerned, however, to seek on several occasions over a weekend period to speak to the respondent midwife, but without success. Eventually, through contacts at the private hospital, he obtained the telephone number of one of the other partners in the practice and spoke to her. He indicated in evidence to the Professional Conduct Committee that he told her the client had been given the scan report to give to her midwife, and summarised to her his findings and concerns, indicating that although the baby had been satisfactory at the time of the scan, it was a potentially high risk situation and that close daily CTG monitoring was indicated. He had added the view that, if the client had not delivered within two or three days, a further scan was recommended to consider in particular the placental blood flow.

Two days later the client went to the same private hospital where the facilities it provided for the independent practice were again to be used. The same hospital midwife attached the client to the monitor, continuing that monitoring for about 40 minutes. The respondent midwife arrived and took over during this time. She (the respondent) subsequently emerged from the room where the monitoring had been undertaken and found both the hospital midwife and the obstetrician (who had performed the external cephalic version) together. She sought their opinion on the trace.

It must be noted that neither the midwife nor the obstetrician had any clinical involvement in the case, did not have full knowledge of the history and were not made aware that the client had a scan 2 days before and of the specialist's expressed concern. The client's clinical care lay with the respondent independent midwife. The hospital midwife indicated that she was very concerned at the abnormal trace she was shown, basing this on the fact that the client was now 3 weeks overdue and in early labour. She contended that what the respondent had decided was 'loss of contact' was, in fact, a significant deceleration. The obstetrician was less concerned, acknowledged that there had been 'dips', but was prepared to accept the respondent's 'loss of contact' explanation. Both advised that the monitoring should be repeated, and offered the client use of the unit's jacuzzi and pool to relax for a period first. The trace resulting from the further monitoring session conducted by the respondent was not seen by either of them.

The client was then told by the respondent that she could go home but should call her if the contractions became stronger. However, as the client was leaving the hospital her waters broke. There was meconium staining which the client described as 'like pea soup'. She returned to the respondent who was still in the hospital. In evidence the client stated that the respondent told her that meconium was to be expected when the baby was so far post-term and that if she went into an NHS hospital they would overreact. She was again told to go home and the respondent would call to see her 2 hours later. The client had not, at this stage, been told to expect anything other than a home birth.

When the respondent arrived at the client's home and examined her she could not detect a foetal heart sound. By this stage the client was having strong contractions. The respondent then called an ambulance to take the client urgently to the NHS hospital with which she had originally been booked. A further scan indicated that the baby had died. The woman was eventually delivered by caesarean section the following day.

Another significant feature of the evidence concerned the matter of whether or not the client was willing to go into hospital. She was adamant in her evidence that she had told the respondent that, whilst they would prefer a home birth, she would gladly go into hospital if there were any problems. She said that the possibility of induction had never been raised with her. She also indicated that, when the respondent subsequently visited her at home at a time when she had some friends present, she (the respondent) left a copy of a report which she had prepared for the Supervisor of Midwives who was conducting an investigation into the events. She said that, when she later read the report, she was shocked at its contents, in that it contained a strong implication that the respondent had made it clear to her and her partner when at the hospital that the labour and birth would have to take place in hospital. Her partner had, she said, immediately telephoned the respondent who had replied that reports had to be written in this manner and that had she not done so she was at risk of being 'struck off'.

Evidence about this report was also given by one of the supervisors of midwives who indicated that, when she questioned the respondent about this matter, the respondent gave her a further document to append to the original report that had annoyed the client. This witness indicated that the impression she had gained from reading the report was that a discussion had taken place with the client in which advice was given. The respondent was now indicating to her that there had been no such discussion and that she had not raised that matter with the client.

Had you been a member of the Committee hearing this case and had heard the evidence given under oath which is summarised here, would you have found the charge that the midwife had failed to properly manage the antenatal care and early labour of the client proved ? If you say 'No', that will conclude the case. If you say 'Yes', you must then go to the next stage and consider whether you would regard this proven fact as misconduct in a professional sense. The 'Code of Professional Conduct' and the 'Midwife's Code of Practice' provide a template against which decisions of that kind are made. What is your decision on that matter?

If you decide that the facts are proved and are misconduct in a professional sense, you must then decide what action to take. Do you, in these circumstances, favour taking no further action or administering a formal caution to remain on the respondent's record for 5 years or removing her name from the register.

Case A4: Head of Midwifery (hospital)/night sister (nursing home)

The respondent in this case was a highly qualified registered nurse and midwife, who, at the time of the offences that led to her appearance in court and conviction was the Head of Midwifery for a major hospital. In addition to her registration status as a nurse and midwife, she also possessed Bachelor's and Master's Degrees, an Advanced Diploma in Midwifery, a Midwife Teacher's Diploma and a Postgraduate Certification in the Education of Adults. However, the offences which led to her conviction and the subsequent hearing before the Professional Conduct Committee related to her second employment as a night sister in a nursing home.

She was the subject of seven charges of professional misconduct, the first of which concerned the theft of drugs (including Co-Dydramol, Distalgesic, Prothiaden and Paracetamol) from the nursing home, the others all relating to the theft (and subsequent use) of cheques from residents in the same home. She chose not to attend the hearing.

The police officer who investigated the complaints and gave evidence in the criminal court was called to give a summary of that evidence and explain the circumstances leading up to the conviction. In essence, this indicated that cheques had been stolen and either used to settle accounts or presented to draw cash, the sum involved being in excess of £2000. The drugs had been found when the respondent's home was searched in the course of the criminal investigation. The police officer confirmed that she had pleaded guilty in court to all the charges which formed the basis of the case before the Committee.

In this case, guilt having been established in the criminal court, the facts of the charges were already established. The Committee's task was to decide whether it regarded those proven facts as misconduct in a professional sense and, if 'Yes' to that, what decision it should then make about her registration status.

Taking account of the template for acceptable conduct provided by the Code of Professional Conduct, would you regard these offences as misconduct in a professional sense? If you say 'Yes' to that, will you leave her with the right to practise in her chosen profession or not? What other evidence would you be seeking to assist you in these decisions?

Case A5: Restoration application (former night nurse, elderly care)

This applicant for restoration to the register had been removed 13 years earlier after she had been found guilty of misconduct in a professional sense. This was as a result of evidence that, on one specific night, when the nurse in charge of a ward for physically frail elderly patients, she had treated those patients in a rough and unkind manner, had shouted at them and verbally abused them, had administered medicines in a careless manner, had been neglectful of their comfort and dignity and had slapped one patient on the face. The applicant did not attend the hearing of the charges that led to her removal. She had been a registered nurse for 6 years at that time.

As a result of its thorough questioning of the applicant the Committee learnt that she had applied for restoration 6 years earlier and that her application on that occasion had been rejected. It also emerged that, with the exception of a period of 4 years when she had not worked, she had held posts as a home help and subsequently as a care assistant in residential homes. References in support of the application had been provided by three former colleagues and a recent employer.

The applicant indicated her awareness that, if her name was restored to the register, it would be necessary for her to attend a 'back to nursing' or 'refresher' course, and explained that her enquiries had revealed that she could not gain access to the course at her local university until her application for restoration had been successful. She explained that she was currently employed, through an employment agency, in a number of residential homes for elderly people, and described the bulk of her work as washing, dressing and feeding the residents. She said that she took this work following the rejection of her previous application, as it seemed that something of the kind would be necessary to convince another Committee of her suitability for restoration.

In response to questioning about the interim period, the applicant said she had unsuccessfully attempted to obtain qualifications as a medical secretary, and had spent some time as a hairdresser before working as a home help and care assistant. She insisted that she was ready to return to her chosen profession, that she had learnt to cope and exercise personal discipline when provoked and added that she had been punished more than enough. She also described the (limited) reading of professional journals she had recently undertaken, and expressed a hope to return to nursing in either a gynaecology ward or an Accident & Emergency Department. She felt that the demands of nursing and the pressures in the workplace would be no different than at the time of the incidents that led to her removal.

Finally the applicant said that she had no aspirations other than to return to nursing and that, if restored, she would do all in her power to justify the committee's confidence in her.

The Committee must choose either to accept the application for restoration to the register, with all that this implies, or reject it. If it chooses to accept the application, the fact she had been removed would be declared to any potential employer seeking to confirm her registration status for a five-year period from the date of restoration. If it rejects the application it would be normal to offer some advice concerning a possible future application.

If you had been a member of this Committee, what would your decision have been?

Case A6: Nurse in care of frail elderly patients in hospital

The respondent in this case was a nurse with 12 years experience since qualification. At the time of the matters with which she had been charged she had held her post in the particular elderly care ward for $4\frac{1}{2}$ years, but for several more years elsewhere in the same hospital.

Through her legal representative, she admitted the three charges of which she stood accused. These were to the effect (1) that she misappropriated over £1500 of money from patients' accounts, (2) that she attempted to obtain a further £350 from the same or similar accounts, and (3) that, in order to perpetrate such misappropriation and the further attempt, she had forged the signatures of four fellow nurses and two nurse managers.

Since the allegations contained in the charges were admitted, it was unnecessary for the Council's Solicitor to call evidence to prove the facts. He did, however, call such evidence as was necessary to enable the Professional Conduct Committee's members to understand the context in which the offences occurred and the financial system that applied. By this means it was explained to the Committee that, following 7 years employment in the hospital, the respondent nurse had been dismissed for 'financial irregularities'.

The 'care of the elderly' ward in which she was employed at the time of the incidents accommodated 30 frail and dependent long-term residents. Personal money was held, for safe keeping, in accounts maintained for them by the hospital's finance department. If a patient required money (for example, to purchase personal toiletries) the nurse designated as the key worker for that patient would complete a form and then have it countersigned by another nurse on the ward staff and subsequently by a nurse manager. The request form was then placed with the cashier in the finance department, following which the key nurse received a bulk sum to cover all the requests for which she had been the originator. The system required that a copy of the request was kept in the 'Cash Request Book' and that when the money was received it should be checked against that book and also entered in a ward cash book.

A routine audit revealed irregularities, and suspicion fell on the respondent nurse. The sum of £1500 which had been misappropriated was made up of six requests in the name of different patients over a three-month period. In each case it was the respondent who had signed the cashier's receipt book, but no consequential entries had then been made in the ward cash book as she had taken the money herself. The investigation revealed that what purported to be genuine signatures of colleagues and managers in respect of the requests for money were all forgeries made by the respondent. The same was true of the further forms which were in the process of being dealt with when the facts related to the first set were exposed.

The respondent admitted the acts of dishonesty and her employers dismissed her and reported the matter to the Council in order that it might consider the question of her future registration status.

Through her legal representative the respondent accepted that these offences did amount to misconduct in a professional sense. That done, he advanced arguments in mitigation to seek to convince the Committee that she should not be removed from the register. He argued that the incidents were isolated and uncharacteristic, that she had learned from the experience, and that there were at the time overwhelming personal problems (since resolved) which led her to behave inappropriately. He also drew attention to her poor health for a substantial period following the birth of twins and her genuine concerns resulting from the illness of one of her children who had needed to be in hospital for 6 months. The fact that the respondent had substantial absence due to illness was confirmed by the nurse manager, but this had consistently been the case throughout her time in the employment of the hospital, and not just prior to and at the time of the offences.

By way of further mitigation, the legal representative drew attention to the good reference provided by the Head of Nursing at the registered nursing home at which she had been employed for several months prior to the Committee hearing, this apparently being written with full knowledge of the facts which were before the Committee.

The respondent nurse herself explained the health problems which had been a feature of her life at the time, her stress then being compounded by marital difficulties culminating in her husband leaving her. At the time of the hearing he had returned to the family. She maintained that she had learned to cope with the stresses of life and that there was no prospect of any repetition of a similar offence or, indeed, any other inappropriate conduct.

Profile evidence given by a manager from the hospital in which the offences occurred was confusing, in that he described the respondent as 'caring and attentive to patients' but also as a 'below average performer'. It was apparent that no manager had ever discussed with her the very large amount of sickness she had experienced over most of the years of her employment in the hospital.

In this case the Committee did not have to prove the facts, as they were admitted. Similarly, the respondent had accepted that the admitted facts were misconduct in a professional sense.

Placing yourself in the Committee's role, faced with this information, would you vote to remove her from the register? If not, would you support the administration of a formal caution which would remain on her record for 5 years and be disclosed to any potential employers, or wish no further action to be taken?

Case A7: Registered nurse employed in a post not requiring a registered nurse

In this case the nurse who was the subject of the charges was neither present at the hearing nor represented in her absence. Evidence was provided which satisfied the Committee and its Legal Assessor that service of the notice of the inquiry to the registered address had been undertaken in accordance with the law in the form of the statutory rules, so the Committee agreed to proceed in the absence of the respondent nurse.

The offences of which this nurse was charged arose from incidents when she was employed as a Care Manager in a residential home for elderly people. This was not a post which, in strict legal terms, required a registered nurse. A registered nurse is, however, in law, able to be called to account by her or his regulatory body, even if the matters complained of occurred in a setting where her registration status was not a condition of employment. One effect of this is that, in terms of the care and treatment of people in her charge, the nurse would still be expected to honour the requirements of her profession's 'Code of Professional Conduct'. The evidence presented made it clear that, although the home was a residential home and not a registered nursing home, many of the residents (age range 70–90 years) did require a certain amount of what can be regarded as basic nursing care.

There were 11 charges before the Professional Conduct Committee. These included such matters as ordering assistants to give breakfast to residents while they were sitting on commodes, being in possession of residents' pension books without cause or permission, failing to call a doctor to examine a resident (a diabetic patient) who had fallen from her bed and suffered injuries to her face and head, failing to notify a doctor when a resident had been given another resident's prescribed medication in error, continuing to administer a medicine to a resident when the prescription had been discontinued and knowingly administering medication prescribed for one resident to other residents for whom it had not been prescribed and not recording that administration. In addition, there was one charge already proved by a criminal court – that of theft of a sum in excess of £2800 made up of money paid in by relatives of residents and some obtained by the misuse of residents' pension books.

Of the 11 charges that had not been the subject of criminal proceedings, the Professional Conduct Committee found ten proved to the required standard. It did so after hearing the evidence of three members of staff of the residential home and its proprietor and taking the opportunity to question each of them in detail. The Committee members agreed that the theft charge and the ten other charges found proved were misconduct in a professional sense, when measured against the Council's expectations set out in the Code of Professional Conduct.

Before retiring to consider its final decision on the case, the Committee heard from the residential home proprietor that the respondent had been in employment at a registered nursing home at the time of her application for a post and that a supportive reference was received from that source and another from the hospital in which she had previously been employed.

Identify now with the members of the Committee with whom rested the decision as to whether the facts and misconduct they have found proved should lead to removal from the register or whether a lesser sanction (or none) should be imposed. They have not had the advantage of meeting the respondent nurse, of questioning her and assessing her demeanour, but that is because she has chosen not to attend. Provided the Committee is satisfied that the notice of the hearing has been served in accordance with the requirements of the law, it can proceed with and conclude a case in the absence of the respondent.

What is your decision? Note that a decision to remove her from the register of nurses would not, of itself, stop her from working in a post such as that in the residential home, but it could prevent her from taking a post requiring a registered nurse in any area of health care.

Case A8: Joint owner/manager (with her husband) of a company providing nursing care and ancillary services to people in their homes

The respondent nurse in this case did not appear at the hearing, but there was sufficient evidence given that the legal requirements in respect of the service of the notice that the hearing was to take place at a specific time and date had been satisfied.

The allegations of misconduct against this nurse which called into question her future registration status were a consequence of her criminal conviction for eight offences contrary to Section 1 of the Forgery and Counterfeiting Act of 1981.

Through the evidence of the police officers who had investigated the events leading to that criminal conviction, the members of the Committee learnt that the sole victim in this case was an elderly lady who had engaged the services of the company for care and other support in her own home. Payment was in the form of cheques which, due to her incapacity, the lady asked the nurse to make out in her presence, but which she then signed. This arrangement operated over a six-month period and, as a result of the consequent alterations to the cheques, a sum in excess of £2400 had been illegally obtained.

The possibility of criminal activity in respect of this matter came to light only when the elderly lady had a problem in respect of her bank account (unrelated to the home care arrangement) and caused an investigation into her account to be conducted. A vigilant member of the bank's staff noticed that the amounts being paid by cheque were greater than the payments required as shown on the invoices. As a result the police were called and the cheques were taken away for examination by specialist handwriting experts. The results of that investigation revealed that the cheques had been written using an ink that could be 'taken off again', allowing subsequent insertion of a different sum. The evidence given by the police witnesses revealed, for example, that £760 had become £960, £1228 had become £1448 and £344 had become £844. All the cheques had been paid into accounts held by the respondent nurse, either in her own name or jointly with her husband.

The forensic experts, on the basis of their study of the writing, considered that the alterations were almost certainly made by the respondent in this case. The police evidence indicated that, when interviewed by them, she had initially denied the charges and contended that the elderly lady was mentally unstable. However, when the matter came before the court, she pleaded guilty to the charges and was, as indicated, convicted of eight offences under the Forgery and Counterfeiting Act. The police evidence indicated that, subsequent to the court appearance, all the money had been repaid to the elderly lady.

The Council's Solicitor indicated that she had been unable to obtain for the Committee any information about the respondent's previous professional history, the only thing being known that she had worked with her husband in this company partnership for some time.

Once again you must place yourself in the role of a Committee member. You have before you details of the offences perpetrated by a nurse who has chosen not to appear before you. You know that, prior to this matter, there was nothing known about her. You know that she has repaid all of the money that she had been identified as obtaining fraudulently. Is that enough for you to feel that you can leave her with the right to practise as a registered nurse, perhaps simply administering a formal caution which would remain on her record for 5 years and be made known to any intending employer who sought confirmation of her registration during that period? Or do you think you can be either more lenient than that or alternatively so tough as to take from her the right to practise?

Like the Committee, you have no opportunity to ask her how she feels about these offences in retrospect, whether she shows remorse, and whether she has grown in professional awareness as a result of her experience. What are you going to do about her?

Case A9: District Nursing Sister/Community Practice Teacher

The respondent in this case was a nurse of almost 20 years experience. The first half of that period had been spent in hospital employment both in the United Kingdom and abroad, and the remainder in nursing in the community in the UK. She had obtained the required specialist qualification for this purpose 10 years earlier and supplemented it through qualification as a Community Practice Teacher 3 years later.

She appeared before the Professional Conduct Committee to answer three charges. These were to the effect that, while employed in the role described, she had:

(1) permitted a video film to be made of a patient which identified her without her written consent, thus failing to promote and safeguard that patient's interests as her regulatory body's Code of Professional Conduct requires;
(2) caused distress to the same patient by permitting a number of people unknown to her to enter the patient's room (in the residential home in which she resided) for the purpose of filming and to call her by a name which was not her own; and
(3) over a period of several months, failed to maintain adequate records in respect of 14 of the patients for whose care she bore responsibility.

The patient who was the focus of the first and second charges had suffered a cerebrovascular accident which had left her with very limited mobility and further handicapped by aphasia. She had also suffered with severe leg ulcers for 2 years. This patient was one of a number who were, with properly obtained consent, participating in a research project involving the use of a new form of dressing.

The conclusion to emerge from many hours of evidence in respect of the first two charges was that a dressing manufacturer wished to have a video made in respect of one of its products and engaged a film company to prepare this promotional film. That company's representative had commissioned a person who was an experienced community nurse but who was also, at the time, professionally engaged in community nursing education, to write a script for the film and to find a suitable patient. He in turn had sought assistance (from his partner in a relationship) to identify a suitable patient and assist in the preparation of the film. This person was the respondent nurse in this case.

Evidence in support of the first two charges was given by a number of other members of the community nursing staff, their managers and the person employed locally as the wound care specialist. There was no dispute that the patient concerned was a participant in a trial of a new dressing product following a long period of her ulcers failing to progress with other products, and that real progress was now being made. Her consent to participate in that trial had been obtained by the more junior nurse who normally attended her and had, with patience and diligence, established an effective means of communication. That nurse had been approached by the respondent (at a very late stage) about access to the particular patient for what she understood to be the video filming of a close-up view of one of her leg ulcers. She indicated that she had assumed that this was known to the community service managers and the wound care specialist, was taking place with their authority, and that there was no further issue of consent since photographs of ulcers of this kind were taken monthly for inclusion in patients' records to record progress or deterioration. The simple proceedings she anticipated was not, however, what occurred.

The oral evidence, and the video film which the members of the Professional Conduct Committee viewed, had clearly indicated that, although the film opened with a view of the patient's leg before zooming in to a close-up of one leg ulcer, it then moved on to a general view of the patient before focusing clearly on her face. It also revealed that (presumably as a gesture towards confidentiality) the patient was throughout, and to her confusion, addressed by a name which was not her own. Under cross-examination the respondent nurse agreed that the video (which she claimed to be solely educational) revealed the patient to be, at times, distressed – even bewildered – by the proceedings, but she stated that she had not sought to halt or interfere with the filming which was going further than she had anticipated because she assumed that the unnecessary material would be edited out.

Although the respondent had argued that she anticipated that the filming would be brief and that her only role would be to introduce the filming team and those associated with them to the patient's nurse and then depart, the various witnesses commented on the fact that she had clearly had her hair done and dressed up smartly for the day, and that she had cleared her diary of her normal nursing appointments for the day so as to be available. They also referred to telephone conversations which they had heard when the respondent was clearly involved in making detailed arrangements with either those responsible for making the film or for commissioning the making of it. The video film also recorded the respondent entering and leaving her car outside the clinic building and in the entrance hall of that building which was her base. It was noted that the residence of the patient selected as 'suitable' for the filming was in a sector of the town which the respondent did not cover, so the patient was not known to her. It has to be assumed that the healing ulcer was the attraction.

One point that emerged as of particular concern from the Committee's viewing of the video film was that, the improving ulcer having been shown in close-up, it then showed the respondent nurse applying a dressing product which was not that being used in the current research programme for which she had consented. The respondent nurse admitted that there was no such dressing in the patient's room and that she took it from her bag to use. The dressing used was a product of the manufacturing company for whom the film was being made, but was not that which was deemed appropriate for this patient at this time. (In later questioning from the Committee, the respondent made an unsolicited statement that she had no hidden or ulterior motive for using the dressing she chose, and rejected the suggestion from a Committee member that she did so because it was that which the film was intended to promote.)

In respect of the charge concerning record-keeping, the major problem identified in a study of the records of 14 of the respondent's patients over a three-month period was that often the only record was brief and in her diary, indicating that a visit had been made. No indication of what had transpired during that visit existed in records held either at the patients' homes or at the clinic base. The respondent accepted that she knew and understood the local record-keeping system, had not challenged it or suggested that any aspects of it were unnecessary, but sometimes had failed to make records of the kind required, the 14 cases cited apparently being examples of this omission.

After due deliberation, the Committee found the facts alleged in each of the three charges proved. It also regarded them as misconduct in a professional sense.

Before retiring to make its final decision in this case, the Committee heard evidence of the significant number of opportunities made available by her managers and which the respondent had grasped to maintain and improve her knowledge and competence. This included a number of conferences, courses and demonstrations directly relevant to her role, as well as others related to professional accountability and ethics. It also learnt through evidence given in mitigation that, at the date of the hearing (and for some months previously) she was employed as a practice nurse in a practice operated by two general practitioners, where she had personally taken initiatives to establish audit and standard-setting and was deemed by her employer to be performing to a high standard.

Through her legal representative the respondent indicated that, at the time of the events that featured in the charges, she had separated from her husband and was undergoing traumatic divorce proceedings with dispute about custody of her son. This, it was argued, conspired to create pressurised circumstances which are not likely to arise again, that the respondent had learned from her mistakes and that she had put her life and career back on path in a constructive manner.

This was a long and complex case. Had you been a member of the Committee which had to consider it, what would have been your judgment? No further action required, perhaps? Or a formal caution which would remain on the respondent's record for 5 years, would be made known to any potential employer during that period, and would be brought forward in evidence if further misconduct was proved before the Committee within that period? Or do you believe that the public interest requires that this person be prevented from practising as a registered nurse?

Case A10: Possession of drugs (not directly related to practice) and theft

The respondent in this case was registered on the part of the register for psychiatric nurses. His appearance before the Committee took place almost 4 years following his conviction in a criminal court for offences under the Misuse of Drugs Act and his further conviction 2 years later for three counts of theft, all of which led to him serving terms in prison which had recently concluded. It was also some 20 months after his release.

The police officers directly involved in the investigation leading to the criminal charges and conviction were called to give evidence of the circumstances leading to the convictions. They described how police officers arrived at a house with a warrant to search the premises, the door being opened by the respondent nurse in this case. The materials found (scales, powder, paper with relevant calculations etc.) led to the arrest of the respondent and another person on suspicion of possession of a controlled drug with intent to supply. In the course of a first interview the respondent expressed shock and said that he had smoked joints on a couple of occasions, but had never used heroin and that all the materials and equipment found belonged to the other person. He therefore denied any involvement. In a subsequent interview he conceded that, following arrangements made by the other person, he had accompanied him to Holland twice to collect drugs and return with them, his part intended to be used to raise money to sort out his financial problems. He claimed that the drugs had only ever been in the possession of the other person. In a third interview, he conceded that this was not true, and that he had been to Holland on his own, the other person conveying him to a sea port for the outward journey and meeting him at an airport on his return. He admitted the importation of heroin (9.36 grammes, with a street value at the time of about £1000) and was convicted on the charge of fraudulent evasion on importation provisions and possession of a controlled drug.

In respect of the thefts, these resulted from reports made to the police by a solicitor who, in making arrangements for power of attorney to be exercised on behalf of one of his elderly clients who was afflicted with Alzheimer's disease, took the appropriate steps to ascertain the contents of her estate. In doing so he contacted National Savings and was informed that £59 000 of National Savings Certificates had, at an earlier date, been cashed and the money paid into a bank account in the name of the respondent. The police investigation that followed had revealed that the respondent had met and befriended this lady when she attended, as a day patient, the hospital in which he worked. She had, during this period, signed forms which were sent by the respondent to the National Savings office and resulted in the sum of £59 000 (the value of three sets of certificates) being paid to his bank account.

The respondent did not challenge the fact that the matters of which he had been convicted were misconduct in a professional sense, and the professional committee so resolved.

Before proceeding further with the case, the Committee was informed that the respondent had some earlier minor criminal history respectively 5 and 7 years before the court appearance on the drugs charges that led to the hearing. The first related to theft from a shop, for which he had been formally cautioned by a senior police officer. The second involved driving with an excess alcohol level, for which he had been fined £150.

To assist the Committee understand the respondent's professional background, the nursing manager who had been the respondent's employer for substantial parts of the period between his original registration and his conviction for drugs offences was called in evidence. His report was of the 'nothing known against him' variety.

In his own evidence to the Committee the respondent contended that all of his problems stemmed from the relationship which he then had with the other person – a relationship that had long since terminated. That man, he contended, had introduced him to heroin without his knowing, and had then got him addicted. He denied any intention of ever selling heroin, but accepted that he had gone to Holland to purchase heroin for the use of himself and his partner. He said that 'the wretched stuff had destroyed his life'. Having served a custodial sentence, he had emerged determined to put his life together and look to the future.

In respect of the thefts, the respondent indicated that he had known the lady in question and her husband for a long time, but with a gap in their contact when he worked in Germany for a substantial period. Contact was renewed when he visited her on his return, and later when she attended the day hospital at which he was employed for periods of time. She was, he said, in her better periods, aware of the deterioration in her mental state, and her main wish was that, at the end, she be allowed her final illness and death at home. The money was transferred to him in order that, when the time came, he personally could look after her. Sadly (he indicated), this coincided with the heroin developments and once the money was in his account the majority of it was spent on heroin rather than to honour his commitments to the lady. This he deeply regretted. In response to questions from the Committee, the respondent said that he had taken no drugs since the day the police entered his home. He had achieved this on his own and received no therapeutic assistance. He added that, by arrangement with an employment agency, he was at the time of the hearing caring for a person with cerebral palsy in that person's own home.

Following a period of deliberation, the Committee's chairman told the respondent that it was adjourning the hearing until a later date, and that for that hearing it wished to receive evidence from his doctor with regard to his current health state, evidence from any professional practitioner (in prison or out) who had assisted him to beat his addiction, evidence from his current employer and any other employer he had served since release from prison and any other evidence which he believed might assist the Committee in reaching its final decision.

At the resumed hearing the respondent presented the requested reports, these including reports also from the Community Drug Team and the Probation Service. All of them supported his own view that he had effectively rejected any use of or dependence on drugs and was, apart from an unsurprising level of anxiety about his registration status, in good health. The report from the agency through which he had obtained employment revealed that the employment was as a care assistant and was not, therefore, strictly a position for which his nurse registration status was required. His client receiving care at home was a mentally alert male adult with cerebral palsy. The respondent served as a 24-hour/7-day-week live-in carer, alternating weekly with another carer. In this role he was overseen by the client's professional social worker who visited frequently and by the care manager/advocate from the social services department. Their reports indicated that a high and effective level of care was given to the client by the respondent, and had been for 18 months since the arrangement commenced. It was apparent from these and other reports that he had a positive and constructive relationship with this client, ensuring that his life was as full as possible.

The Committee noted that, from the time of his release from prison, the respondent, in seeking employment, had always been totally honest about his past. It was against that background that one of the Directors of the agency interviewed him in depth and decided to provide him with work with the client described above. The respondent indicated that, beyond work, he spent his time caring for his disabled and now wheelchair-bound mother or on his own in his flat. If he was removed from the register he said he would continue in his present or similar caring roles. If his name remained on the register, after a few more months, he would seek to re-enter psychiatric nursing, first seeking advice and assistance about the kind of re-entry programme he might need to attend before seeking employment.

This is the person and these the facts on which the Committee had to pass judgment. Had you been one of them, what would your decision have been? The events were serious, but were now a long time ago. Does this affect your judgment? Has the rehabilitation you would have sought possibly occurred already? Would removal from the register now have more to do with punishment than public protection? These are the kind of questions the Committee have to wrestle with in a case like this. So should you.

Case A11: Conviction for conspiracy to murder

The nurse who was the subject of this case was neither present at the hearing nor represented in her absence. Evidence was presented to confirm that the notice of the hearing had been served in accordance with the law on this matter. The charge, based on the conviction in a criminal court some time earlier, was that the respondent had been convicted upon indictment of the offence of conspiracy to murder and had been sentenced to serve 2 years imprisonment, that sentence on appeal being reduced to 12 months of which only 4 months was to be served and the remainder suspended. This was clearly a light sentence for an offence of this magnitude, indicating that the court must have accepted that there had been provocation.

Evidence was given by the Police Officers who were involved in the investigations which led to this conviction. This indicated that, in response to a report of an aggravated burglary, they went to a house. Their findings suggested initially that a burglary had occurred, entry having been gained through a window. One of the persons present in the house was an adult male who was in bed surrounded by blood-stained bedding, it appearing that he had been attacked with knives. Also present was his wife (the respondent in this case) and a mentally handicapped eight-year-old girl in an adjacent bedroom. From their examination of the scene and enquiries of nearby residents, the police officers concluded that this was not primarily about burglary, but its purpose had been an attack on the injured man.

Pursuing that line of inquiry, suspicion initially fell on another family member who, it was believed, had previously been harmed by the injured man. On further investigation, the police officers formed the view that perhaps the family had colluded to arrange for the man to be attacked and possibly killed. In the course of a further interview, the respondent confessed to conspiring with others to have her husband killed.

In respect of the injuries suffered by the injured man, these were described as primarily injuries to the hands and forearms that would be sustained in fending off a knife attack, but there were also two injuries to the chest wall which was not penetrated. As for the background to these events, it appeared that, over the period of their nine-year marriage (the second for the respondent) there had been turbulence and persistent problems. The three children of the first marriage, who had initially stayed with their mother, had left her home as a result. The respondent wanted a divorce, but her husband did not agree.

The police found a witness who had been approached by the respondent with the thought of 'doing away with her husband' and offered money to assist. It appeared that, shortly after that conversation, and by chance, the respondent's daughter met another young woman (a person who had been abused by her own father) who, after hearing of the circumstances and what they were thinking of doing about it, suggested that she should kill the man on behalf of the family. This apparently led to a series of meetings at which plans were laid in considerable detail, the 'burglar' even being appraised of which of the stairs should be avoided as it creaked. Some of the defendants in the case stated that the man was to be drugged so that he would not waken during the attack, but it was never established whether this actually happened.

On the night planned for the attack the respondent had retired to bed where she lay beside her husband. The young woman who actually carried out the attack told the criminal court that a window was left open for her to gain entry and that she then turned off the electricity and disconnected the telephone. She also stated that she had then changed her mind about carrying out the attack, but the man woke and at that stage she did attack him.

There were four people involved in the conspiracy – the respondent who was the man's wife, her daughter and son-in-law and the young woman. The police officers indicated that, after the first interview, the respondent had cooperated fully with them and clarified all the elements of a very complex case. As indicated, the respondent was not present of her own choice. In these circumstances the Professional Conduct Committee members read the written statement which she had provided for the Preliminary Proceedings Committee to consider when deciding whether or not to forward her case for hearing.

This case was not related to professional practice as a nurse, but is quite properly being considered as it raises profound questions about a person who is a registered nurse. At the time of the offence the respondent was not employed as a nurse but in an administrative capacity for a local college. You are a member of the Professional Conduct Committee. What decision are you going to make about this respondent's future registration status? You have not had the advantage of meeting and questioning her, but neither had the committee members.

Case A12: Registered midwife – practice standards and record-keeping

The respondent in this case was a registered midwife of more than 17 years standing who had been employed in either a full-time or part-time capacity for all of that time, always on night duty, by the unit that eventually dismissed her from employment and brought the complaints against her to her regulatory body. The charges arose from her care of a woman in labour and the eventual delivery of that woman's baby in a very poor condition when she was on night duty in the labour suite of a hospital maternity unit. They related both to her alleged failure to observe appropriate standards of care and deficiencies in her record-keeping. She had only the one woman in her care on the particular night.

The evidence given indicated that the respondent had been alone with the woman and her partner from midnight until she was delivered of her baby at approximately 4 AM. The midwifery manager had received reports from other midwives who came on duty the following morning which expressed their concern about what they regarded as particularly inadequate records in a case in which the baby had been born in a poor condition which might, in their view, have been the product of inadequate monitoring. Having examined the records, the manager shared their concern about both the quality and the timing of the records made by the respondent (feeling that they may have been made in retrospect rather than contemporaneously) and the apparent quality of her monitoring of the patient.

It appeared that the the monitor which the midwife was using for part of this period was faulty in that the CTG trace was only being recorded intermittently (and infrequently) and, while this was happening, no records of any significance were being made during the 2 hours before delivery. Such CTG traces as had been produced by the faulty monitor had been 'lost' and were not, therefore, available as evidence. Evidence given by other witnesses indicated that there had been another monitor available for the respondent to use.

In her own evidence the respondent midwife indicated that she had taken over the care of the woman at midnight and had initiated monitoring from that time. She had discarded the first monitor she used as it was not operating properly, but had not reported that fact. She said she first experienced problems with the next monitor and was not obtaining a trace from about 2 AM. Thinking that the problem may have been with the fetal scalp electrode she had attached, she changed it, but after correct operation for only a few minutes that also only provided a trace only intermittently. She stated that she left the room in search of the unit's small portable sonicaid monitor, but found that it was in need of charging, so she initiated that and moved on. She then searched for a Pinard stethoscope, but failed to find one. The evidence of other midwives was that there was always a Pinard stethoscope available in the labour suite, but that it was used only rarely because the monitors were routinely used.

In the absence of either of these alternative monitoring methods, the respondent indicated that she opted to discard the fetal scalp method and instead use an abdominal transducer. This still left her with the problem of a machine producing only an intermittent trace. She chose to be content, telling the Committee members that she so decided because 'it was only the graph that was the problem' and she had audible and visible indicators from the machine. She had made no record of the information this provided for her, and she stated in response to a question that she did not normally make any records other than the CTG trace.

The midwifery manager stated that her expectations of a midwife in this predicament would be that she change the monitor, change the fetal scalp electrode again, use abdominal monitoring, do everything to ensure that the baby was being properly monitored and call for more senior help and support. When questioned by members of the Committee, the respondent said she did not consider changing the monitor again because she believed she was receiving adequate information. She contended that she was adequately monitoring the fetal heart. In respect of such record entries as were made, it became clear from questioning of both the respondent and other witnesses that the bulk of the entries for the two-hour period prior to delivery were made some 3 or 4 hours after delivery and when the baby had been transferred to the special care baby unit. Her case was that another midwife who entered at the time of delivery, seeing that the baby was in a poor condition, took charge of her and also of the records. She said that she only caught up with the notes and was able to make her records related to the delivery when she found them in the special care baby unit. This did not really address the question of the absence of any recorded entries for a substantial period prior to delivery. It became clear as the case proceeded that what every other person regarded as inadequate in respect of records the respondent saw as adequate, and she repeated her statement that she normally kept no records other than the CTG trace. The records she made in retrospect did, however, include entries for five specific times during that period. She had not, even then, however, complied with the local policy in that her entries were not signed and had to be identified by her writing.

Given that her original education and training as a midwife predated the use of monitors and that she had been on permanent night duty, the Committee was anxious to learn how she came to be instructed in the use of fetal heart monitors. The respondent's answers they found worrying, in that she described an arrangement whereby, when new equipment was received, it was demonstrated in the daytime and 'one of the day staff would show the night staff and it was handed down'. She denied ever having any training in the use of monitors or instruction in the interpretation of monitor traces. She also accepted that she had made no request that this deficit be remedied. The further the questioning went the greater was the Committee's concern about the use of equipment which was not understood.

The Committee found the facts alleged to be proved to the required high standard and, despite the persuasive address from the respondent's representative, considered these facts to amount to misconduct in a professional sense.

At the next stage of proceedings the Committee heard from the person who had, for a substantial part of the respondent's employment in the hospital concerned, been the Director of Nursing and Midwifery. From this the Committee learned that the respondent was on record as having attended a fetal monitoring event run by the manufacturer of the sonicaid equipment 7 years earlier (that is 9 years after she commenced employment there as a midwife) and a one-day course on monitoring and interpreting CTG traces in the same year. The witness said that the respondent would have had the opportunity to be instructed on the use of the equipment, as would any other midwife, but there was no record of it having happened. She had also attended the required refresher course for midwives three times during her period of employment, but there was no evidence of her having attended any other internal or external events for the purpose of professional updating. In answer to the question from a Committee member 'So are you telling us then that you were satisfied that Miss X was competent in the use of fetal heart monitors?' the same witness responded 'I am saying that she would not have been allowed to work on the labour ward had she not herself said that she was competent'.

In his final speech in mitigation, the respondent's representative grasped upon the now exposed weaknesses in the management of the unit as exemplified by some of the evidence referred to above. He emphasised repeatedly that nobody had questioned her knowledge or competence or at any time indicated that her record-keeping failed to meet the required standard. Only the Committee's penetrating questions had, he claimed, made her aware of her failures. He contended that the respondent had learned a hard lesson and that the Committee could be assured of her future standards. He advised the Committee that, at the date of the hearing, having completed the counselling course in which she was a participant at the time of the incidents, she was now giving her time as a volunteer counsellor for a unit whose clients had drug and alcohol problems.

There in outline you have the picture that emerged over several hours of evidence and examination. It is apparent that the unit, its management, and the arrangements it had in place to ensure the competence of its professional staff, were less than perfect. That does not alter the fact that, as the Code of Professional Conduct makes clear, the individual practitioner bears a personal accountability for her actions or omissions.

What is your decision to be in this case? Do you leave this midwife with the right to practise in her chosen profession, or do you take away that right by removing her name from the register?

Case A13: Fraud related to professional practice

The respondent in this case was an enrolled nurse (i.e. a second level registered nurse). She was not present at the hearing. A letter had been received from the respondent stating that she would not be attending, so there was no doubt about her being aware that the hearing was taking place. The charge followed a conviction in a criminal court for fraud and attempted fraud, for which she had been fined £250 and required to pay compensation of £1225. She had pleaded guilty in court.

It was explained to the Committee that, having been placed for nursing duties by a major nursing agency, she completed and posted to the agency 23 time sheets that were fraudulent in three respects. First, she claimed to be a first level registered nurse, and thereby gained additional remuneration. Second, she claimed for more hours than she had actually worked. Third, she forged the signatures of seven clinical nurse managers to authenticate her claims for payment. Her actions went undetected for about 3 months, during which time she had been paid £1225 more than that which was properly due to her. The attempted fraud followed the same pattern, but was discovered when a further ten claims were being processed for payment. Had these been cleared, a further excess payment of £699 would have been made. The Committee agreed that the facts which had been proved in the criminal court did amount to misconduct in a professional sense.

In her absence there was little additional information available to the Committee. It was told, however, that she had been placed in nursing positions by the same office of the same agency for several months 4 years earlier, but then went to live and work abroad. When she returned she contacted the agency to say that she was again available for work. From that point until her fraudulent conduct was discovered her contact with the agency was only by telephone and post.

What is your view of these events? It is apparent that slack administrative procedures at the agency allowed her fraudulent actions to go undetected for some time. Had the agency taken steps to confirm her current registration status when she returned to them after a four-year break, the first element of her fraud would have been quickly detected. Their inefficiency does not, however, excuse her fraud. Does this offence require her removal from the register or a lesser sanction?

Case A14: Restoration application of nurse removed from the register 3 years previously for unfitness on duty due to alcohol, and other offences

This applicant for restoration to the register had been removed from the register 3 years earlier after three charges of misconduct had been proved against him. He had, at the time of removal, been a registered general nurse for 10 years and a registered psychiatric nurse for 12 years. The offences that led to his removal occurred in a ward for 30 elderly mentally ill patients. In this setting he was proved to have been under the influence of alcohol while on duty; using foul and offensive language in the presence of patients, their relatives and fellow members of staff; and leaving the ward without adequate nursing staff cover.

The Professional Conduct Committee members were told that the committee which took the 'removal' decision heard evidence to the effect that, when coming on duty to take charge of a shift, when receiving a report from staff on the previous shift, he interrupted them with statements littered with foul language. He was said to have been 'animated', speaking with a loud voice and smelling of alcohol. It was said that he used foul and crude language to patients, and about fellow staff in the presence of patients and their relatives. By way of illustration, it was said that he had asked an elderly female patient if she would like to have sex with him, and made sexually offensive remarks about a more junior member of staff in the presence of other staff. Finally, some 2 hours before the shift was due to end, he suddenly left the ward, saying he was unwell, leaving it understaffed. He had been in charge, but did not take any steps to hand responsibility for the ward to any other member of staff.

At the original hearing, after the facts had been established and proved to be misconduct in a professional sense, the Committee learnt that, at the time when he commenced his employment at the hospital at which the incidents occurred, the fact that he had suffered with an alcohol problem was made known, but it was believed that things were under control and he was not then drinking. Some time prior to the events that led to his dismissal from employment and subsequent removal from the register, his problem was seen to have returned and he was referred to the hospital's Occupational Health Department. The professional staff of that department authorised his return to duty under supervision. There was another incident which led to him being given a final warning, but this was not heeded.

At the hearing which was considering the restoration application the members heard that, since removal, the applicant had worked first in a small retail static and mobile shop and subsequently at a petrol filling station. Seven months prior to the hearing he had been engaged in a community care project as a project worker. He explained to the Committee that this meant that he was working with former patients of the local psychiatric hospital who were readjusting to life in the community and described the one-to-one support and assistance to develop life skills that this involved. In addition he was giving some of his time voluntarily to assist at a drop-in centre for persons with mental health problems.

In respect of the alcohol dependence, he stated that the history of his problem was a very long one, but that he had now avoided alcohol for more than 4 years. He said that this was the longest period of sobriety he had ever had as an adult. Though very confident, he continued to attend Alcoholics Anonymous twice a week for his own purposes, but was clearly pleased that others now sought him out as their sponsors rather than it having to be the other way round. 'Giving something back' had clearly become important to him. His personal life (not surprisingly strained by his previous condition and conduct) was on an even keel again, and he was living happily with his wife and two daughters.

His retrospective view of the conduct that led to his removal was one of potent self-criticism. What was he doing to try to reassure the Committee that he would not again behave in so appalling and unprofessional a manner? First, in his own words he provided an impressive statement of the attitudes and standards which professional nursing requires. Second, he indicated that he was not complacent, that he would go on taking things a day at a time, each day reinforcing his determination not to return to the use of alcohol because he knew his vulnerability.

He had no immediate plans to re-enter nursing practice if restored, but was exploring the possibility of a part-time degree course first. In respect of being abreast of current nursing issues, he had been assisted in this by his wife who was a registered nurse in current practice and ensured that he read all the relevant documents that she received. In another aspect of his life, he had completed the relevant training and qualified as a football referee, which he saw as providing him with another useful outlet and a further opportunity to make a contribution to his community.

In his final statement to the Committee before it had to make its decision, he again emphasised his disgust at his past conduct which had put not only him but his profession to shame in the eyes of those who witnessed it or had otherwise become aware of it. For this he expressed profuse apologies. He reiterated his rejection of alcohol and his determination, if restored, to uphold the standards of the profession. The picture he presented of himself was supported by reports and references from people with full knowledge of the facts.

These are the facts on which you must now make a decision. Remember you are not now judging the original incidents. They were proved and that led to his removal from the register because it was believed that such an action was necessary in the public interest. Now you have the equally difficult task of deciding whether this is a person to whom you can again give the right to practise in his chosen profession. Is this man suitably rehabilitated? Do you accept his application and then remind him in the strongest possible terms of his responsibilities and accountability? Or do you reject the application? If you take the former decision, the fact that he has been removed and later restored will be kept on record for 5 years and declared to any person who seeks to confirm his registration status. What are you going to decide?

Case A15: Misappropriation of medicines from hospital workplace and possession of cannabis and amphetamine

The respondent in this case was a young man who, having successfully completed his pre-registration education and training, had registered as a psychiatric nurse 3 years before the discoveries that led to his dismissal from employment and referral to his profession's regulatory body.

The first charge that he faced related to the fact that he was found to have in his possession a small quantity of tablets (analgesics, tranquillisers and sedatives – 53 tablets in total) which he had stolen from the ward in which he was employed. This was an acute psychiatric admission ward of 30 beds, invariably with a high occupancy. The second charge stemmed from his possession of 1 gramme of amphetamine sulphate and a small quantity of herbal cannabis for his personal use. He admitted the facts stated in the charges and that these matters were misconduct in a professional sense.

The evidence presented by the investigating police officers explained that his possession of these items came to light when, acting on information received, the police obtained a warrant authorising them to search the respondent's room in the hospital residence where he was then residing. Police officers arrived on the ward (on which, at the time, he had been working for 15 months) and explained the nature of their visit. They cautioned him and asked if he was in possession of any controlled drugs. He replied that he was not. He then went with the police officers to his room. As a result of the authorised search, the officers found a plastic container in which were the tablets that became the subject of the first charge. He stated what the tablets were, and admitted that he had stolen from the ward. He was detained on suspicion of theft and possession of controlled drugs. At the request of the police, the respondent then accompanied them to the ward in order that they could examine the contents of his locker. There, in a sports bag, they found the items that became the feature of the second charge. Of the amphetamine he was said to have commented 'It's speed' and of the cannabis (0.232 gramme) 'It's grass – I forgot I had it.' He stated to the police that he had those items for his personal use and, when taken to the police station, freely admitted theft of the tablets and possession of the other items. That is a summary of the police evidence.

After due consideration by the relevant officials, no criminal proceedings took place in respect of these matters. The hospital authorities conducted their own inquiry and subsequent disciplinary proceedings, as a result of which the respondent was dismissed from employment and reported to the Council so that his future registration status could be considered. It was stated in evidence that, in the course of the employer's first inquiry hearing, the respondent stated that he took the tablets from the ward over a period of about 4 weeks. He said that he did so for his own use because he was having difficulty in sleeping. When asked why he had resorted to self-medication and whether he had sought professional help, he said that he had experienced difficulty in getting an appointment with his doctor who was a long distance away. The respondent accepted that the information given was accurate in most respects, simply adding that the amount of amphetamine sulphate was only 0.4 g.

In his own evidence to the Professional Conduct Committee, the respondent explained that he did not have general health problems, but that at the time pressures in his life had been building up for several weeks. He said that the pressure of work was great, that he had personal and relationship problems and was having a problem with sleeping. His doctor, he said, was 15 miles away (near to the hospital from which his ward had been moved), and because of the pattern of his shifts he had not been able to get an appointment to see him. Before he had been able to fulfil his intentions in that respect the police had arrested him with the known consequences.

In response to questions, he added that the analgesics were taken because he was experiencing sinus and tooth problems and that he did not know why he had taken so many tablets from the ward, since he had used only five or six. He said that it was an extremely silly thing to do and emphasised that he did not have a drug problem but had always had difficulties with sleeping which became a 'problem' during this short period. He added that his personal problems were now resolved and that he was living with his girl friend. He had not sought nursing work pending this hearing, but was working in a factory temporarily.

In respect of the nature of the work pressures at the time, he said in answer to a Committee member's questions that it was a very busy ward, that there were usually more patients than there were beds, that many patients really needed one-to-one nursing but there was not the staff to provide it, and the result was that, if you tried hard to deliver good care as he did, you were 'stressed out'. He again emphasised that his personal circumstances had changed and that after his dismissal he had benefited from great support from family and friends. He added that he enjoyed psychiatric nursing and working with patients, believing himself to be good at his job, so he would hope to return to nursing if the Committee made that possible.

In order that the respondent's career background and the context in which he was practising at the time of the discoveries could be better understood by the Committee, a senior nurse manager was called in evidence. He explained that the respondent had been taken into their employment immediately after becoming registered. The acute admissions ward in which he was employed from the outset was relocated from the hospital at which the respondent began employment to be part of a psychiatric unit within a large general hospital some distance away. It was explained that, as a junior staff nurse, he was part of a team and that there would normally be more senior qualified nurses on duty. It was accepted by the witness, however, that there were times, particularly when more senior post vacancies occurred and new appointments awaited, that the respondent would have to bear more responsibility and sometimes be in charge of the acute admissions ward. This had been the situation for some of the weeks preceding the events featured in the charges.

The witness indicated that the hospital had an Occupational Health Department. The managers had never felt cause to refer the respondent to the service. Staff members could attend of their own choice and the service was entirely confidential. He also indicated that there had been no previous disciplinary problems with the respondent and no cause for concern about either his attendance at work or his performance. The respondent had attended the various events made available by his employers for professional development and had generally shown a desire to be professionally aware and competent. The respondent accepted the general accuracy of the evidence given by this witness.

In his final statement to the Committee in mitigation, the respondent stated that he had not known that an Occupational Health Unit accessible to staff by self-referral was available at the hospital. In respect of the offences which he had admitted, he emphasised his regret and his realisation that his actions were stupid when he had friends and family to support him. He emphasised that he was not using any drugs and would not think of ever doing so in the future. He expressed the hope that he would be able to return to nursing the mentally ill, because he believed he had the ability to serve them well.

These, in summary, are the facts that you should now consider. Does the public interest require the removal of this young nurse from the register or will some lesser sanction be sufficient? Do you get the impression that he has learnt from the experience and is unlikely to renege on his promises, or does a significant risk remain? You know that his attendance and performance at work was deemed satisfactory. What is your judgment on this respondent?

Case A16: Community nurse – theft from elderly patients

A 35-year-old community nurse was the subject of a hearing by the Professional Conduct Committee on charges of misconduct arising out of incidents in the course of her work. The hearing was a consequence of the nurse having been convicted in a criminal court of the theft of sums of money from patients she had been visiting in the course of her professional duties.

It emerged from the evidence that the nurse was considered to be caring and skilful. It was also said that she was liked by her patients and formed extremely good relationships with them and any relatives and friends who visited them in their homes at times she was calling. In short, she was liked, respected and above all trusted.

Since the nurse had been convicted in a criminal court and the court had imposed a suspended prison sentence, that formed the basis from which the Committee had to operate. The official documents certifying the conviction were submitted as proof of the facts alleged. The evidence heard related to the circumstances leading up to those facts.

That evidence indicated that the nurse had a fairly average caseload in terms of numbers, but one that contained an above-average number of elderly patients. In the course of her visits to those elderly patients and the need to go to various drawers and cupboards for clothes (etc.) the nurse came to be aware of the places in which some of them were keeping substantial sums of money in bank notes. For example, one had wads of notes in pockets stitched to the sides of her mattress, while another kept them under her clean underclothes in a drawer.

There were six patients involved in the charges. The time came when each of them was either going into hospital as a planned admission or moving house. In each case the nurse volunteered to go (in her own time) to help them pack. It was in the course of this activity that some of the accumulated money was apparently taken. In the case of the five going into hospital, the nurse (writing in her professional capacity rather than as a friend assisting them to pack) wrote notes to accompany them which indicated to the ward staff that the old ladies were confused. Faced with that information the hospital staff had not regarded the matter seriously when the ladies, over their first 2 weeks as inpatients, complained about their lost money. It was only when a relative of one of them did believe the patient and made representations to the district nurse's line manager that the matter was investigated. The details of that investigation need not trouble you, but you need to know that in this way a little over £2000 had been stolen from six elderly, dependent patients.

The facts were established by the certificate of conviction. The Committee then had to determine whether they regarded those facts as misconduct in a professional sense. Look at the Code of Professional Conduct to see what parts of the Council's advice to its practitioners are relevant and then decide whether you would regard those facts as misconduct. The Committee did, and then proceeded to hear evidence as to the previous history of the respondent and any mitigation before retiring to make its decision.

The respondent had chosen not to attend, not to be represented in her absence and not to submit any mitigation for the consideration of the Committee. In order to hear something of her previous history the Committee heard evidence from and questioned her former nurse manager. This witness, speaking from experience over several years and on the basis of monitoring visits done with the respondent, told the Committee members that she had always found her to be skilful and competent, with an apparently good relationship with patients and their relatives. She had clearly been shocked by the fact that such allegations had been made and proved against a nurse she had previously believed to be a person of integrity and was distressed at having to give her evidence.

You are now the Professional Conduct Committee. Accepting that the facts have been proved and regarded as misconduct, what is your judgment? Consider also whether any people in this case in addition to the respondent need to be the subject of comment when the Chairman announces the Committee's decision in public, and what lessons emerge for your work setting.

Case A17: Fracas in psychiatric unit – assault of patient

A 30-year-old registered mental nurse appeared before the Professional Conduct Committee as a result of an incident that was alleged to have occurred shortly after he came on duty to commence his shift at 1.30 PM. The charge he faced was to the effect that he had ill-treated a patient by striking her and that he had responded inappropriately to the patient's request for attention.

In the course of the evidence received from the patient and several members of the staff, the following picture emerged. The nurse (who became the respondent in this case) had been off duty for the previous 2 days. On the day in question he came on duty to commence a later shift. He was to be in charge of the ward, it being one of three in a psychiatric unit of a large district general hospital. He received a hand-over, in the course of which he was made aware that the patient who became involved in the incident (a woman of 50 years of age) had been admitted the previous day with a depressive illness. He recalled that he knew her slightly from an early brief period as an inpatient for the same reason. He was not told of any problems to which she had been seeking to draw attention or of any requests she had made for assistance during the morning and was given no indication to suggest that she had not received (in her view) an appropriate response to her needs and requests.

Having received the hand-over report, the respondent nurse, accompanied by a student nurse, commenced the administration of medicines. They were doing this from the doorway of a small clinical room in which the medicine trolley was securely locked and stored when not in use. The respondent nurse had the trolley located just inside the room and patients were coming to the doorway to receive their prescribed medication. The student was in the clinical room, the respondent nurse and trolley therefore barring his way but not his vision. The nurses' station was located in the corridor and near to the clinical room so that, on emerging from the door of the clinical room it was necessary to deviate slightly to the left to avoid the end of the desk unit.

When prescribed medication was being administered to other patients, the patient in this case came to the trolley (she said in her own evidence that she was fairly angry) and demanded something to treat a headache. She was told by the nurse that there was no appropriate prescription, that she should go away and that he would arrange something for her later. What he did not know (but what became clear from later evidence) was that she had been complaining of a headache and asking to be given something for it during most of the previous shift.

The administration of medicines was nearing completion when the patient returned, vociferously and bluntly complaining of her headache and shouting that she had waited 'all bloody morning' for some tablets. That said, she suddenly thrust a hand towards the containers of medicines in the trolley. The nurse's response to her action was to quickly slam down the lid of the trolley against the patient's hand and lower arm. Her already existing anger being fuelled by this further reaction to her, the patient flailed her arms as if to strike the nurse and produced a stream of expletives indicating what she thought of him. At this stage it was alleged and the evidence indicated that the nurse punched the patient, striking her on the jaw, as a result of which she fell to the floor in the corridor. At that stage he quickly pushed the trolley back into the clinical room and rushed out into the corridor only to crash his thigh against the end of the nurses' station and himself fall to the floor. The evidence indicated that he rose and called the student nurse to assist him and that they together picked the struggling patient up and carried her into the nearest room with beds which ran off the same corridor opposite the clinical room. The intention was to place the struggling patient on the nearest bed, but it transpired that the bed wheels were not locked and as they leant against the bed to do so it ran away from them and the patient again fell to the floor.

The evidence demonstrated that at this point another patient, having shouted the question 'Are you teaching Doris karate?' joined the action by picking up a chair and striking all those involved. Things escalated further with some other patients joining in. In less than 2 minutes the scene had moved from one patient crossly demanding something for her headache to something approaching a full-scale riot. Other staff on the ward and those from other wards in the unit were required to restore order to the scene.

The respondent nurse, while admitting that the patient may have been struck, insisted that it was only a necessary action taken in self-defence as she flailed a series of blows generally in his direction and that he had certainly not punched her on the jaw. This view was contradicted by the evidence of the patient, the student nurse and a domestic assistant who had also witnessed the events.

The facts alleged were therefore denied but were found proved to the standard of proof the law requires (the Committee must be satisfied so that it is sure). That brought the Committee to the stage of the hearing where it must determine whether, when looked at in context, the facts constitute misconduct in a professional sense. What is your decision on that point?

The Committee resolved that the proven facts did constitute misconduct in a professional sense and therefore had to receive any evidence in mitigation and of the previous history of the respondent before making its final judgment on the case. No character evidence was produced by the respondent or his representative. In providing previous history of the respondent a professional manager from the health authority indicated that, in his 2 years of employment with that authority, the respondent had been a generally satisfactory employee, their main concern focusing on the point that he showed little imagination, took no initiatives and was generally reluctant to accept change.

You must now put yourselves in a position of the members of the Professional Conduct Committee and decide on the judgment appropriate to this case which you find it necessary to make, reflecting the profession's global responsibilities to the public. You might also consider what other persons contributed to this incident and their degree of culpability relative to that of the respondent nurse and also ask yourselves whether any particular concerns need to be drawn to the attention of the employing authority as a result of this incident.

Case A18: Registered midwife – diabetic patient and elective caesarean delivery

An experienced midwife appeared before the Professional Conduct Committee of the UKCC alleged to be guilty of misconduct in a professional sense. The charges stated that she administered Monotard and Actrapid by injection to a diabetic patient without following the correct procedure and when those drugs had not been prescribed. The allegations were denied. The respondent was present and represented by a barrister so the evidence of the witnesses was thoroughly tested in cross-examination.

The patient was admitted to hospital for an elective caesarian section operation. It was normal practice to admit such patients on the day prior to operation and to starve them from midnight. The patient was an established diabetic who had been taking insulin at home in the form of Monotard 40 units and Actrapid 16 units daily at 7.30 AM. Admission records were made by a student midwife and a junior doctor, both of whom noted in their records the patient's established insulin regime.

The operation was performed the next day. On that day a senior doctor prescribed 500 ml of 10% dextrose with potassium chloride and 10 units of Actrapid insulin each 6 hours. Later that day the dose of Actrapid in each 500 ml of 10% dextrose was reduced to 5 units. Both prescriptions were properly recorded in the prescription sheet for intravenous fluids and additives.

The respondent was on night duty on the relevant ward for the night following the patient's operation. Another midwifery sister was in charge of the whole maternity unit for that night. On her round at 10 PM she discussed the patient's management with the respondent and enquired of her what treatment the patient was receiving and how often blood sugars should be done. She recalled asking the respondent whether she knew what the normal level was and receiving a negative answer. She told the respondent to contact the house officer. The same witness also recalled (1) asking the respondent if the patient was to recommence her insulin injections in the morning and the respondent saying that she was; and (2) visiting the ward later when the respondent told her that she had contacted the house officer and had been told the normal blood sugar reading using the Reflomat test.

This sister and other witnesses described the arrangements for prescribing and administering drugs in the hospital. There was a form headed 'Prescription Sheet' with a section for drugs to be given once only and another for continuing prescriptions. This document showed the local policy to be that drugs were to be administered only in accordance with prescriptions written on that prescription sheet. Records of drugs administered were kept on a 'Drug Recording Sheet', which contained two statements to the effect that those administering drugs should refer to the prescription sheet for the details of the dose and route of administration. In addition there was a further prescription sheet for 'Intravenous Fluids and Additives'. The procedure document for the health authority was widely available and a copy was in the drugs trolley.

At 7.30 AM on the morning after the operation, the respondent administered 40 units of Monotard and 16 units of Actrapid although this had not been prescribed by any doctor and there was no entry concerning it on the prescription sheet. She made a clear entry on the 'Drug Recording Sheet' that these drugs had been given. At the change of shift the day sister received the night report from the respondent and, at 7.50 AM, was told by the respondent that she had given the patient her 'insulin dose of 40 units Monotard and 16 units Actrapid'. The day sister commented that the patient was not yet eating and was continuing to receive intravenous therapy of 'dextrose and potassium chloride and 5 units of Actrapid in each 500 ml'. The respondent said that she had followed the doses stated in the patient's notes. It was pointed out to her by the day sister that those entries in both the clinical and nursing notes were part of the admission history and not instructions or prescriptions for that insulin to be administered as an inpatient. Contrary to local policy, no other member of staff had been involved in checking or observing the administration of the drug.

The Council's solicitor called the patient and six other witnesses, all of whom were cross-examined by the barrister on behalf of the respondent and questioned by the Committee members. At the end of the 'Did It Happen' stage of the hearing the Committee found the allegations proved to the strict standard of proof required.

The respondent's barrister then argued that the Committee should not regard the facts proved as misconduct because (in her view) bad practices prevailed in the hospital, the drugs procedure was poor, the prescriptions were 'dismal' and the error was a 'one-off' in a long career. The Committee did, however, find the facts proved to constitute professional misconduct.

The Committee then received information about the respondent's previous history and the material that she wished to submit in mitigation. The midwifery manager for the health authority said that she had known the respondent for 7 years, though not particularly well, having only recently stepped into a role that gave her closer contact. She said that the midwife had first been appointed as a special care sister because she had experience in that field and had obtained the Midwife Teachers Diploma. She moved to the main midwifery unit 6 months after appointment because she needed to do part-time night duty to fit in with her husband's studies. The witness confirmed that, during the respondent's employment she would have encountered diabetic patients on the maternity unit with reasonable frequency since they were cared for in the normal maternity wards. The witness summarised the respondent as being 'a pretty average midwife' and indicated that such criticism as there had been related not to her professional work but to her general attitude towards her work.

In mitigation from the respondent it emerged that, prior to undertaking a Midwife Teachers Diploma, she had been active in teaching student midwives and in planning and organising their courses. While working on night duty and seeking to organise her life to fit in with her husband's studies, the respondent had also been a mature student and had obtained a BA degree at polytechnic. She had continued her studies and obtained an MA and was now undertaking studies for a PhD. Although well qualified academically and continuing her advanced studies, the respondent indicated that she hoped and expected to use her nursing and midwifery qualifications again, though not necessarily in the clinical setting. Three letters of testimonial in support of the respondent were submitted.

Put yourself in the position of the members who served on the Professional Conduct Committee. You have before you a highly qualified professional nurse and midwife. You have proved her guilty of misconduct in a professional sense for a fairly basic error which she did not recognise to be such and which occurred when all the available information and a question raised by her superior should have helped her to avoid it. She is not in current nursing or midwifery practice but has declared to you her intention to use again the registration which she wishes to retain.

Consider also whether other people contributed to this occurrence and should be made the subject of criticism in the announcement of the decision and what lessons emerge from this case that might be applied in your own work setting. Indeed, ask yourself 'Could this happen where I work?' and 'What do I need to do to avoid it happening?'

Case A19: Health visitor – caseload size and record-keeping

A 43-year-old health visitor (RGN/RHV) appeared unrepresented before the Professional Conduct Committee facing 17 charges alleging misconduct. Two charges alleged failure to keep a record of official mileage for which reimbursement was claimed, four alleged failure to keep health visiting records in respect of visits, two alleged failure to record the results of hearing tests, two alleged failure to record the results of developmental screening, three alleged failure to record on primary record cards the results of phenylketonuria (PKU) tests, two alleged failure to forward immunisation consent forms to the relevant sections and the final two alleged failure to forward data sheets to the Pre-School Health Section.

The respondent admitted the facts but required the evidence to be heard before the Committee adjudicated upon the matter of misconduct.

The evidence revealed that, 3 years after she had taken up the health visitor post in question (having moved from a similar post with the adjacent health authority), the respondent was on holiday. At this stage, there having been some difficulty with a disparity between caseloads, a count was undertaken with a view to reallocation. As the respondent was on leave and had not completed her part of the count the nursing officer obtained access to her records. She discovered discrepancies. Together with a colleague, she then carried out a detailed investigation. This revealed considerable problems in respect of the records. Some had no entries. Some development test reports had not been entered on the records. Some vaccination and immunisation consent forms had not been passed on. When the respondent's diary was checked it was noted that she had not kept any record of the mileage for which she had sought reimbursement. When these matters were put to her by her manager she could give no explanation.

In her evidence to the Committee the nurse manager (to whom the respondent had been responsible) defined the basic duties of the health visitor as 'To home visit mothers and babies, antenatally and up to 5 years old, and then school nursing and teenagers if necessary; to perform routine development screening, and offer advice and support to the care of mothers and young babies'. She told the Committee that four health visitors worked in her area, with average caseloads of 400 children aged 0–5 years. The witness also told the Committee that it was local policy that diaries be used to record visits, trips, lectures given and mileage travelled. Other policies related to developmental assessments on a 9–18–36-month plan, hearing tests to be performed between 7 and 9 months, and the recording of PKU test results. In respect of immunisation an offer was made to all parents, and where they consented the consent form was sent to the Vaccination and Immunisation Department who sent an appointment for the child to be taken to the appropriate clinic.

It was against her statement of the role and the local policies that the nursing officer had found the respondent wanting, in that there were primary record cards of some two-year-old children with no entries, some three-year-old children with no entries after 9 months, cards with no PKU results recorded or attached or with no hearing test and/or developmental test entries made. A quantity of PKU reports were found in a drawer. It should be noted, however, that the same witness had called in the cards annually for a check on the distribution of work, and had not previously observed the deficiencies since she simply did a count of the cards, and not an examination of even a sample of them.

In response to the questions from the Committee the witness said that the HV service was organised on a GP attachment basis where a patient moved into an HV's area but retained her GP in another area by arrangement, and that the annual review was of workload (including time spent at antenatal classes, parentcraft classes, clinics, GP work, and health education) and not just caseload. It also became clear that health visitors completed a monthly return as to how many hearing tests they had done in the period, but this (she said) did not contain names and did not serve as a check on individual HV record cards.

Pressed by a member of the Committee about her responsibility to monitor the work of her staff and her manner of doing it, the witness said that health visitors were highly trained practitioners, so she would not do planned monitoring visits, but if there was ever a complaint she would follow it up and then perhaps look at a random sample of record cards. Since she had received no complaint about the respondent she had done no such sampling. The witness also confirmed that in the light of this case the whole system of monitoring, management and induction had changed, and that although the plan was to undertake formal appraisal of health visitors annually, this had never happened with this employee in 4 four years with that authority.

In her own evidence the respondent drew attention to the fact that the nurse manager's evidence had failed to indicate that it was required that each HV keep a birth book with details of each child born in or moving into the area, that it also should be checked by nurse managers, and that in that book there were columns for recording PKU results, hearing and developmental test results, and the move to school or out of the area. Her records in that respect were complete. She challenged the nurse manager's statement about the monthly return regarding hearing tests, stating that there were individual sheets attached to the monthly return, and that these indicated whether it was a first or second test, the result, and whether the case was being referred on to the community physician. She similarly and quite effectively challenged some other aspects of the nurse manager's evidence.

The respondent confirmed that she had not maintained the records referred to in the charges, but that she was contesting that she was guilty of misconduct on certain of the charges since she had made records of those matters in other documents which the health authority also required her to keep. It was clear that she could speak in a detailed manner about the children and families which could only have been the result of frequent visits and great interest in them.

In spite of the respondent's submission, the Committee considered the facts in respect of all charges to be misconduct. The hearing moved to the stage where evidence in mitigation or aggravation is heard. The director of nursing services gave details of the respondent's record in general nursing, industrial nursing and health visiting prior to taking the post in which the charges arose. Her career appeared to have been exemplary. The reference from her previous HV post referred to some tension with colleagues, but also to her strength as a leader and her leadership qualities. This witness said that she had met the respondent on a few occasions only, but had found her intelligent and stimulating. She referred to her innovative ideas and approach, and told the Committee of a course she had run for her colleagues to demonstrate counselling techniques which was 'excellent and received the highest praise from all who attended'. She went on to say that when she interviewed the respondent about the gaps in her records she failed to grasp the enormity of her failure or to provide an explanation, so she dismissed her from employment.

Pressed by the Committee, the same witness agreed that one of her interviews had been at the request of the respondent who had brought with her a critical analysis of herself which exposed her problem regarding paperwork and documentation, and stated that as a result she instructed the nurse manager to 'chase her up for her monthly statistics'.

In her own address in mitigation the respondent spoke of the practical problems she had overcome as a single parent to train as a health visitor, but that she bore those burdens to take up the career of her choice. She accepted responsibility for her failures, but felt that the response to them had been excessive since she had worked satisfactorily as an HV in other places. She had, on taking up her post, found that relationships between the various professionals involved (two GP practices operating from the same base) were 'stormy' and stated that she had tried to be a mediator. Although there was a part-time clerk to do some clerical work for the HVs, because the previous staff had not used her she (being conscientious) had filled her time with other health centre work which she then could not shed. In any case, her skills did not include shorthand or audio typing. Attempts to get the nurse manager to come to talk about these problems had failed. She said that the general attitude of the managers was that 'If you are finding it difficult you are not good enough for the job'. She gave details of a number of innovations which had been a feature of her practice, and which were clearly impressive.

A clinical psychologist who attended as a friend of the respondent confirmed the problems of the health centre and the many difficulties arising from staff attitudes and staff changes and spoke of the high level of concern and high standard of care the respondent provided for her clients. Numerous testimonials were also submitted.

The Committee members felt that they had before them a committed, articulate, innovative health visitor, but one who also needed the sort of manager who would help keep her feet on the ground and ensure that basic tasks were done before advancing into new territory, while still encouraging innovation.

You know that the facts are admitted and are seen as misconduct. What will you now do by way of passing judgment?

Case A20: Patient abuse and management failure

Three experienced nurses (one enrolled nurse, one ward sister and one nurse manager) from a general hospital ward were the subject of a joint hearing before the Professional Conduct Committee which stretched over 2 long days. All denied the allegations made against them.

The enrolled nurse was alleged to have struck one elderly patient, to have treated another patient in a rough and unkind manner, and to have made derogatory remarks of a sectarian nature to a teenage patient who was hospitalised far from home.

The ward sister was alleged to have failed properly to investigate two of those matters which had been the subject of complaints made to her by the teenage patient's mother and a student nurse respectively.

The nurse manager was alleged to have failed properly to investigate the alleged rough and unkind treatment, and in effect to have colluded with the ward sister in a cover-up when that allegation was relentlessly pursued by the concerned student nurse.

The cases began to emerge for consideration only when that student nurse wrote to the statutory nursing bodies, her local representations seeking investigation of and action concerning the enrolled nurse's alleged reprehensible conduct having seemingly failed. By this time a staff nurse in her first post (with the same employment authority), she wrote to the Council to allege misconduct against the above-mentioned three practitioners, and also a senior nurse manager. The latter's case was not forwarded for hearing by the Preliminary Proceedings Committee, but she did find herself called in evidence.

When the Council's solicitor began to investigate the matters alleged, two more former student nurses (by then staff nurses) volunteered evidence of the 'striking' incident, as did the young patient. The two nurses and another colleague provided evidence about the atmosphere on the ward.

The witness who originated the allegations told the Committee how she had seen the enrolled nurse repeatedly poke an elderly patient and physically throw her into a chair. She said she was taken aback as she had never seen anything like it before. She was troubled by what she had seen, but found it difficult to raise the matter with the sister, as the two sisters and enrolled nurse of that ward seemed to constitute an inner circle from which all other staff were excluded. After 3 weeks of agonising (overlapping with studying for finals) she felt she could keep silence no longer, told the enrolled nurse she intended to complain to the sister about what she had observed, and did exactly that. She said that the sister told her she would investigate the matter and come back to her.

The combination of moving from the ward, studying for final examinations, eventually passing and becoming a staff nurse pushed the matter to the back of her mind until she overheard the conversation of some student nurses (who had recently passed through the ward in question) which led her to believe that comparable incidents were still occurring. As a result she wrote to the sister, reminded her of the incident she had reported and the date, reminded her of the undertaking to investigate and report, and courteously asked what transpired.

She did not receive a reply from the sister or the nurse manager, but from the senior nurse manager. That letter said that the matter had been investigated and resolved, but gave no information. The young staff nurse wrote back to express surprise since she was the complainant and she had not been asked for a statement, and again courteously asked the nature of the investigation. The response she received again provided no information, but suggested she make an appointment to see the senior nurse manager. This she did, and when she went to that appointment after night duty she was faced by the senior nursing officer and the nurse manager. She received no answers to her questions, but felt she was faced with pressure to accept that the complaint had been investigated and resolved, and to pursue the matter no further. It was following that interview that she wrote to the Council to allege misconduct.

Corroborative evidence about the atmosphere on the ward came from the other student nurses. One said 'I felt the sisters and enrolled nurse were like a little unit on their own and the rest of us were outsiders'. Two of those witnesses also provided evidence of the alleged striking incident. The young patient and her mother provided evidence of the derogatory sectarian remarks, which in turn had led to a second complaint to the sister which it had been alleged had not been investigated.

In respect of the nurse manager, it was alleged that she had accepted the sister's conviction that the roughness/unkindness had not happened, finding this possible because she also had known the enrolled nurse for some years. It emerged in evidence that two undated documents which purported to indicate that an investigation had taken place subsequently appeared in the enrolled nurse's file, but the fact remained that the complainant had not been asked for a statement.

After nearly 2 days of evidence for and against the allegations the Committee found all of them proved to their satisfaction. There seemed to be absolutely no reason why the witnesses should go to such lengths and personal inconvenience to support fabricated stories. Having found the allegations proved, the Committee considered them all to be misconduct in a professional sense.

At the mitigation/aggravation stage of the hearing the Committee learnt that, once the original allegation letter to the Council had been copied by the complainant to the director of nursing services, earnest efforts had been taken to investigate and take action in respect of the three respondents.

None of the three had been dismissed from employment, but the management had taken steps in respect of each of them which were brought to the attention of the Committee. In respect of the enrolled nurse, the employers seemingly recognised that she had become institutionalised and her judgment impaired through working for so long in one specific ward, and had arranged a refresher course following which she was relocated to another ward. Evidence was received that her performance was being closely monitored in that work situation, and that she was performing well. Excellent references were received about her performance in general, and it was believed that she was normally regarded as a kind person.

In respect of the ward sister, it was brought to the attention of the Committee that her employers had arranged for her to undertake a development programme following which she had returned to her ward where it was believed she now recognised her failure to handle properly the matters which were the substance of the charges, and had earned the confidence of her director of nursing services.

In respect of the nurse manager, the more senior managers, recognising that she had been thrust into a nursing manager role without preparation and at a time when no senior nursing manager was in post, had provided her with management training, enabled her to attend a variety of seminars and study days, and actively involved her in drawing up policies in the areas in which they believed she had demonstrated a deficiency. Again it was brought to the attention of the Committee through references that she was tackling her post with enthusiasm, and had demonstrated a new initiative in embarking on part-time studies for a degree.

The members of the Committee obviously had to feel concern about each of the three practitioners whom they had found guilty as alleged, and guilty of misconduct in a professional sense. The enrolled nurse they saw as having abrogated her responsibility of care, in that she handled patients in a manner alien to the standard of practice expected of a qualified nurse. In addition, she had failed to satisfy the requirement of the Code of Professional Conduct that she accord respect due to the customs, values and spiritual beliefs of a patient. In respect of the ward sister, they saw her as having on two occasions, demonstrated a failure to take seriously and investigate properly complaints made to her, the substance of which were very serious. She had failed to satisfy a prime responsibility to ensure that the standards of practice on her ward were maintained to a high level, and failed to monitor what went on in the ward. The members were in no doubt that the proper investigation of complaints is a component of fulfilling the responsibilities of a ward sister, and any views held by the person about the competence and standards of a member of staff should not influence her when complaints are brought. In respect of the nursing manager, the members deplored the fact that she had been thrust into the nursing manager role without appropriate training or induction, and without appropriate support, and believed that her employers had placed her in an impossible position. Although she had responded extremely unwisely to a situation which had developed, it was felt that she had been placed by her employers in an extremely difficult position.

See yourself as a member of the Professional Conduct Committee. You have before you three persons who have, in their respective ways, failed to behave appropriately, and you have found the allegations against them (which they denied) to be proved and have regarded them as misconduct. You have also heard something of the management context within which they offended, and the things said in mitigation. Now you must decide whether, in respect of each of them, you would administer a formal caution to remain on the record for 5 years or remove from the register or take no action apart from giving advice on standards of conduct.

In addition to that, ask yourself whether this could happen in the place in which you work or for which you have a managerial responsibility, and use it as a stimulus to examine your own practice.

Case A21: Operating Department – error and concealment

A registered general nurse who was a very experienced operating theatre sister came before the Professional Conduct Committee of the UKCC to answer an allegation arising out of an incident in the course of her work.

The circumstances of the case were that, in an operating theatre for which she had responsibility and where she had been a scrub/instrument nurse for a sequence of cases, there had been a long and busy day. The final case on the list involving an abdominal operation for an elderly gentleman was completed only at the very end of the day shift, and the sister cleared the instruments away and put them into the automatic washer within the theatre suite, told the two members of the night staff who came on duty that this had been done, and requested that they remove them later. The evidence was that the two nurses on night duty had subsequently removed the set of instruments from the washer and laid them out on a tray to check, at which stage they found that one Dunhill forceps was missing from the set. They stated that they boldly labelled the tray to this effect in the event that they did not see the sister (the respondent nurse in the case) personally in the morning.

As it transpired they did see her and told her that the set was one instrument short and that they had therefore kept the incomplete set together on a tray which was boldly labelled to this effect, and which they now drew to her attention. It was said in evidence that the sister's reaction was that it could not be as they described, since she was always meticulous about her instrument checks. Having drawn attention to the matter and completed their shift of duty, the night nurses left.

The regulations covering that theatre suite required that, should it be necessary to draw an instrument from the reserve stocks to make up a set, this should only be done by calling in the nurse manager responsible for that set of theatres, or the sister/charge nurse acting up in her absence. This did not happen in this case, since the evidence showed that the sister had subsequently found the set was indeed deficient through the absence of the Dunhill forceps, and drew a replacement from the reserves without the involvement of any other person, and without informing either any member of the surgical team involved or her superiors.

Three weeks later the patient died from something unrelated to the surgery which he had undergone, but in circumstances requiring a post-mortem examination. In the course of the post-mortem a Dunhill forceps was found in the patient's abdominal cavity, as a result of which some enquiries ensued about the circumstances of the operation. The information set out above in respect of the missing instrument and the replacement from the reserve stock then emerged.

Faced with this situation the decision of the employing authority had been to dismiss the theatre sister from employment and to report the matter to the statutory bodies as a result of which the Professional Conduct Committee hearing was taking place. The allegation (which was to the effect that the sister had failed in her responsibility when it was reported to her that an instrument was missing, and acted to conceal the incident) was denied, but was proved on the evidence. It was also argued by the respondent and her representative that the Committee should not deem that which they had found proved to be misconduct in a professional sense.

Consider how you would have responded had you had to determine whether these now proven facts constituted misconduct in a professional sense. Consider also your reasons for whichever decision you make.

In the event the Committee determined that it did regard those facts as misconduct, so the case progressed to the stage at which evidence in mitigation or aggravation is heard. It emerged that the respondent had worked in theatre nursing continuously since her registration some 12 years earlier, had been employed as a theatre sister in a number of famous hospitals in this country and overseas, and was if anything regarded by her last employers as having been almost obsessional about her instrument checking to the neglect of some of her other responsibilities as a sister. It also emerged that the practice in the theatre suite in question was that, whilst the swabs were subject to a check involving several persons, responsibility for the instruments had rested with the instrument nurse alone, though the latter practice had been changed in the light of the case.

It also emerged that, very soon after dismissal from her employment, the respondent had obtained a post as a theatre sister in a private hospital some 50 miles away. It appears that they were so delighted when approached by a very experienced theatre nurse that they had not taken up a reference from her previous employer. Although she had come to the hearing with an excellent open reference concerning her competence as a theatre nurse from her new employers, it also became clear in questioning that the reference was written without knowledge of the incident which led the respondent to be before the Committee.

Now place yourself in the role of a Professional Conduct Committee member again. What decision will you make?

Case A22: Newly qualified nurse – dilemmas on night duty

A newly qualified registered sick children's nurse, aged 21 years, came before the Professional Conduct Committee as a result of incidents occurring in the paediatric ward where she was employed as a staff nurse on night duty.

On completing her training successfully she found that there were no staff nurse posts available in the area she knew, so she had no alternative but to study national advertisements. She made application to an authority several hundred miles from her familiar setting, and travelled to take up her post.

Although taking up a post in her own paediatric speciality she was in all other respects a stranger in a setting in which staff turnover was very limited. She had an induction programme of 3 days duration, following which she was placed in charge of a paediatric ward on night duty. The incident which led to her dismissal and to her subsequent appearance before the Committee occurred only a few weeks later.

On the night in question she was in charge of a busy 25-bed ward with a number of very ill children (for example, three in cubicles had meningitis), with support staff of one pupil nurse and one auxiliary, and with knowledge of the fact that the night sister covering her ward was not a specialist paediatric nurse.

At approximately midnight she became concerned about the condition of a particular baby and decided that some suction was indicated. She took the baby to the treatment room, only to find that the fitted suction equipment was not operating. Fearing that the baby was deteriorating, she carried him quickly to another location where there was some portable suction equipment and again attempted to pass a tube. She had difficulty and believed this might be the result of congestion in the nasal and upper respiratory passages. She decided (a) to administer 2 drops of Otrivine to each nostril (knowing that it was not prescribed), (b) to call the doctor, and (c) to call the cardiac arrest team, which she did in that order. She also repeated her attempted suction, this time successfully.

When others arrived they determined that there had not been an arrest, and that the baby was now satisfactory. The doctor for the paediatric unit was not told by the staff nurse that she had given Otrivine drops, but as it happened wrote a prescription for such.

The staff nurse did not give the first prescribed dose but signed as having done so because she had given them prior to the prescription. This troubled the pupil nurse who subsequently mentioned it to a senior person, and an investigation ensued. In the course of that investigation it was noted that a few nights before, while not having the official authority to do so, the staff nurse had responded to pressure from a junior doctor to give some intravenous additives for her, and had quite clearly recorded that she had done so.

She was therefore charged with misconduct for giving an unprescribed drug, for not reporting that she had done so, for not giving the first prescribed dose, and her part in the matter of the IV additive. She had been dismissed by her employers.

The respondent did not deny the allegations, and was willing to accept that they could be regarded as misconduct, but told the Committee that on the night in question she genuinely thought that the baby was going to die and that she panicked, her experience of managing a crisis of this nature being none.

The Committee received good references from her training school, and a report from the Nurses Welfare Service about her difficult family background and early departure from home. It also noted that she had not wasted her time since dismissal and while waiting for the hearing, but had taken up social work training at a polytechnic, whence came good reports and references. She had helped fund her course through part-time auxiliary/assistant work in both health and social work settings.

The facts are admitted. Would you regard those facts as misconduct? If so what judgment will you pass on this young woman who has made it clear that, though preparing for a social work qualification, she wishes to retain her nurse status and possibly work at some future stage in a role that bridges both spheres.

Case A23: Abuse of access to patient's residence and property

A 50-year-old registered mental nurse appeared before the Committee to answer two charges arising out of matters relating to her work. She had been employed at a day centre which was a joint health and social services venture staffed by a full-time specialist social worker, two full-time nurses (one a charge nurse and the other being the respondent employed in a deputy charge nurse capacity), and several community service volunteers. In addition to their work in the centre the two registered nurses were also responsible for some home visits in the locality, particularly in respect of patients who attended the day centre.

One such patient around whom the charges revolved was an elderly lady who had become incapable of managing her own affairs and was the subject of a Court of Protection Order. She attended the centre and was also visited by the staff at home, and it therefore became well known to them (as to the specialist social worker on the team) that the patient (who lived alone) was having to move from a large family house into a much smaller dwelling. As a result of this it was going to be necessary for her to dispose of a considerable amount of furniture, having first decided what items she would retain for her smaller accommodation. Arrangements for an auction of the spare furniture were in the hands of a solicitor who was an agent for the Court of Protection.

It was alleged that the respondent nurse in this case identified some items of furniture which she would like to have for herself, and engaged in some form of barter both in face-to-face meetings with the patient and in telephone conversations. It was also alleged that, the day before the patient was to move to her smaller dwelling, the respondent made urgent arrangements for her husband to remove a number of items of furniture and instructed a young man who was one of the community service volunteers to accompany her husband with his van to the house, ensure that he was given directions and assist with the removal of the furniture. It was further alleged that the community service volunteer was given £100 in cash to give to the patient in exchange for the furniture, he also being required to indicate that more would follow later. He was subsequently given another sum of between £35 and £40 to pass on to the patient. Further to that, it was alleged that, when some time later, the story about the 'exchange' of a number of items of furniture (including a dining table and eight chairs, a chest of drawers and a plant stand) became known to the director of nursing services on receipt of a letter from the social worker, and when he in turn arranged to take the matter up with the respondent, the respondent sought to persuade the community service volunteer to state a false story in order to clear her.

It is important to note that the community service volunteer was a young man who had moved very far from his home in the North East of England because of difficulty in obtaining employment, that the event involving the exchange of furniture for money happened very early in his time at the centre, and that though recruited through social services he spent much of his time working at the centre with the nurses or going with them on visits where his assistance was required. With no previous knowledge of the world of work he had deemed it logical to do as the respondent instructed him in respect of the removal of the furniture, but he absolutely refused to be party to the fabrication of an untrue story, the essence of which was that he tell the director of nursing services that the furniture had really been for him to transfer to his parents who were existing in deprived conditions with very little furniture, and that the money was a loan to him from the respondent to pay for it.

The allegations were strongly denied by the respondent through her representative, but on the evidence of the community service volunteer and of the director of nursing services, were found proved. The evidence of the latter was that of an interview with the respondent in which she had made it clear that she knew the patient's affairs were under the control of the Court of Protection and that this meant she was incapable of managing her own affairs and particularly her financial affairs. He indicated that he had elicited that she had known it was wrong to deal directly with the patient, and that she had made no attempt to deal through the solicitor.

The evidence of the community service volunteer was that the furniture was not his, had not been wanted by him, and that the money which exchanged hands was not money borrowed by him from the respondent in order to buy the furniture. He said that the respondent had raised the question of the furniture with the patient when he was present on a community visit, that the patient had said the furniture had to go to the sale rooms, and that though more substantial figures were at first mentioned the respondent had persuaded the patient to drop the price for all the items of furniture in which she was showing an interest to about £140.

The allegations having been found proved on the basis of the evidence and in spite of the respondent's denial, the Committee was addressed by the respondent's representative to the effect that these matters should not be regarded as misconduct. However, recognising the Code of Professional Conduct as the backcloth against which allegations of misconduct are judged, the Committee deemed those matters which they had proved to be clearly contrary to the introductory paragraph to the Code, and in particular to clauses 1 and 9, the latter of which states that each nurse (etc.) shall:

> Avoid any abuse of the privileged relationship which exists with patients/clients and of the privileged access allowed to their property, residence or workplace.

Consider first whether you would have regarded these proven offences as misconduct in a professional sense. Then accepting that misconduct was proved, consider what judgment (had you been a member of the Committee) you would then have made.

Case A24: Intensive Therapy Unit – failure to monitor effectively

A 25-year-old woman employed as a junior sister in an intensive therapy unit of a district general hospital appeared before the Professional Conduct Committee to face allegations which arose from the death of a patient in the unit.

The people who brought the allegations accepted that the patient's prognosis was poor in any case, but still believed that the circumstances raised serious questions about the safety of the practitioner who became the respondent.

In the intensive therapy unit in question it was discovered that the alarm on a particular type of positive pressure ventilator sounded with great frequency if it was used for mandatory assisted respiration at a rate of six respirations per minute or less. The matter was not drawn to the attention of the nurse managers of the hospital concerned, nor to the manufacturers of the equipment. Instead an *ad hoc* practice was developed in the unit (to which some of the medical staff including consultant anaesthetists were party) to switch off the alarm if the rate for which the machine was being set was six per minute or less.

This practice seemed to have been pursued without any unsavoury consequences for some months. However, on one particular day when there were three registered nurses on duty in the unit and only one patient, the patient's condition deteriorated to such a degree and in such a way that, had it not been switched off, the alarm would have sounded and called nursing staff to give urgent attention. The patient died.

At the Professional Conduct Committee the fact that the *ad hoc* practice of turning the alarm off had developed was not challenged – indeed, one consultant anaesthetist told the Committee that he had often come into the unit and heard the alarm sounding and took the necessary action to disconnect it because the problem was with the machine and not the patient. In support of such an action he argued that the alarm was meant to be an aid to human observation by a suitably qualified person and not a replacement for it.

The Committee had no difficulty in finding that the sister in question had turned off the alarm on the machine, but were faced with something of a dilemma in that one of the other trained staff on the ward at the time had subsequently performed required observations on the patient and had not turned it on again.

At the mitigation stage of the proceedings it became clear that the nurse in question had a previously unblemished record.

See yourself as a member of the Professional Conduct Committee. In particular, considering this case against the background of the UKCC Code of Professional Conduct, would you have regarded the proven action of this sister as misconduct in a professional sense? If so would you have then felt it necessary to remove her name from the register or not? In addition consider what lessons this case might have for your own practice and the settings in which you work.

Summary comment on case studies

The case studies set out for your consideration in this chapter represent but a small sample of the actual cases considered by the Professional Conduct Committee in the course of any one year. They are, however, broadly representative of the type of charges (whether stemming from complaints from the professional practice setting or following convictions in criminal courts) that the Committee has to consider each year.

Since the UKCC became the single regulatory body for the nursing, midwifery and health visiting professions in the United Kingdom in 1983, there has been a noticeable consistency in the types of charges that have come before the Committee each year. That Council's published statistics for the year April 1995 to March 1996 reveals that the six most frequently occurring '*practice-related*' charges were:

- Physical/verbal abuse of patients 30.25%
- Failure to keep accurate records or report incidents 10.14%
- Failure to respond to patients' needs 9.60%
- Unsafe clinical practice 6.88%
- Other abuse of patients 6.52%
- Drug-related incidents 3.99%

In respect of charges that were *not* related to professional practice (usually following criminal convictions), the three most frequently occurring charges were (1) misappropriation of drugs, (2) convictions for theft and (3) offences of violence.

In respect of '*practice-related*' charges that were found proved and considered to be misconduct in a professional sense, and where a decision was then made to *remove the person's name from the professional register*, the six most frequently proven offences were:

- Physical/verbal abuse of patients 29.20%
- Unsafe clinical practice 8.27%
- Failure to keep accurate records or report incidents 7.75%
- Other abuse of patients 6.20%
- Theft from patients 4.39%
- Failures in drug administration 4.39%

When misconduct had been proved and a decision to remove from the register made in cases where the offences were not related to professional practice, the most frequently occurring three charges were again misappropriation of drugs, convictions for theft and offences of violence.

Chapter 14

Professional Accountability Case Studies: 'Aspects of Accountability and Ethical Practice'

A short series of studies illustrating dilemmas experienced by practitioners in the course of their professional practice (to be considered in association with Chapters 1, 2 and 7)

Unlike the cases in Chapter 13, the practitioners involved in these studies have not been the subject of any complaint alleging misconduct, so they have not been subjected to consideration and judgment by any professional committee. Instead they are based on actual telephone calls and letters made by practitioners faced with a dilemma and seeking assistance. The assistance given is that of listening, allowing the practitioner to talk the issue through, and assisting her or him to arrive at their own considered decision.

They ask you to put yourself in the shoes of the person who was actually faced with the dilemma described and to consider what your answer would be to two important questions.

(1) What do you consider to be the appropriate professional response in the situation?
(2) What do you think you would actually have done?

It is important to remember that, in matters such as these, there is often no one correct answer. It is down to the professional judgment of the individual concerned.

Comments (rather than answers) concerning these cases are provided in Appendix 1. I recommend that reference be made to that section only after each study has been read, considered and discussed.

Study B1: Police request for information

A young man – victim of a very serious assault – has been admitted to the resuscitation room of a busy Accident and Emergency Department of a hospital. The injuries suffered by the patient as a result of the assault include multiple skull and rib fractures that are commensurate with him being severely beaten and kicked.

On arrival at the department the young man was accompanied by his father and sister, both of whom had witnessed the attack. They were extremely distressed and frightened. They state that the attack was for entirely racist motives, and that they are afraid not only for the safety of their relative (the patient) but for their own safety in the community in which they lived.

Following initial resuscitative treatment the patient has been transferred urgently to the operating department for surgery. At this stage two police officers arrived in the department and approached the Department Sister who was also the nurse in charge at the time. She had been personally involved in the care and treatment of the patient while he was in the department.

Having realised that it is not possible for them to speak to the patient, they ask the Sister some questions. In particular, they explain that a man is in custody 'assisting them with their enquiries' in connection with the attack and that, in order to pursue their investigation, they need information concerning the injuries suffered by the patient. They ask her to provide that information. Further to that, they ask her if they may see the patient's relatives who they know to be still in the hospital in order to ask them questions about the incident and their opinion of the condition of the patient as a result.

In considering or discussing this case study, remember the two questions set out in the introduction to this chapter.

Study B2: Caring for a confused elderly patient

A nurse employed in a residential nursing home arrived on duty one morning, knowing that she was to take charge of the nursing team in the home for that day. The particular home was one that provided long-term nursing care for elderly patients.

She was concerned about one of the elderly residents who, over the previous few weeks, had become increasingly confused. Twice in the last month she had been found wandering around the gardens outside the home in a very distressed and tearful state. In the past she had, on occasions, enjoyed a brief walk outside, but had always done so only when one of the nursing staff or one of her visiting relatives had been able to accompany her. On the recent occasions when she had been found outside on her own it was evident that she could not remember leaving the home or understand why she was outside and what she was doing there.

The nurse was particularly concerned as she arrived for duty on this day because she has been told that, on the previous day, the lady had wandered far beyond the grounds of the home and was found, by a helpful member of the public who personally returned her to the home, meandering down the middle of a road in the nearby town. As on the previous occasions which had caused less concern, once back in the home the lady had quickly become aware of her surroundings, was lucid, and promised that she would not go outside unaccompanied.

In view of the previous day's event, the nurse was concerned that the lady would not remember her promise, and that she might wander again and endanger herself. She was aware that this resident is a very private person, never spending time in the lounge or other communal areas, so it is difficult to always be sure where she is. The staffing numbers make it impossible to have a member of staff available to observe this one resident all of the time. The nurse wonders how she can respect this lady's freedom in what is now her home, yet ensure that she comes to no harm as a result.

The same two questions posed in the introductory text need to be considered.

Study B3: A terminally ill patient and her will

An elderly woman was admitted to a hospital ward, knowing herself to be terminally ill. As a patient she proved particularly demanding. First, she was dissatisfied with the facilities available to her and asked the charge nurse to arrange to move her to a private room. This he did as soon as a room became available, but her relative satisfaction was short-lived. She continued to make many more requests. More blankets, more pillows, special food, a different private room with a larger window, and so on. The requests seemed endless, but the charge nurse, mindful of the patient's terminal illness, did his best to accommodate them and ensured that the nursing team did all that they possibly could to make her comfortable.

Then one day the patient asked to see the charge nurse privately. She explained to him that she now wished to make a will and asked him to make the necessary arrangements for her. That said, she began to thank the charge nurse for all that he had done for her. She apologised for being so demanding and asking for so many things and stated that she now wished to make amends and say thank you. To that she added that she had no living relatives and that all her friends had died, so she now intended to leave all her money to the charge nurse. She was insistent that there was no one else to whom she could leave the money and asked the charge nurse to respect this, her last important wish.

The charge nurse is now faced with a dilemma which he had never expected to face.

How would you respond in this situation? Once again, consider these circumstances against the two key questions.

Study B4: Consent for surgery after premedication

Picture this scene. You are a nurse working in an operating department and are about to scrub for the first case in a busy list. The first patient on the list is a woman aged 29 years who has been diagnosed as having a cancerous growth in the bowel.

The notes reveal that this young woman (the patient) has been earning her living as a model, but has recently been considering making a career change as she feels that she is getting too old to continue with that work for much longer. That, however, is her source of income at the time of her admission to hospital. The operation planned for her, and which has apparently been discussed with her, is for resection of part of the bowel. This is the operation described on the operating list and that for which the patient has signed a consent form.

The surgeon now arrives in the operating department where the nurse is preparing the required pack and instruments for the operation. He states that he is now of the view that the patient requires not just a resection of part of the bowel but a total colectomy. This means that she will inevitably awake from the operation with an ileostomy.

The patient now arrives in the anaesthetic room accompanied by her husband. She has been given a powerful premedication, but is still able to converse with her husband, telling him how very relaxed she feels. The surgeon at this stage states that it will be preferable for the colectomy to be performed as soon as possible. He asks you to obtain a new consent form and present it to the patient to sign for the operation he is now intending to perform. He is aware that the patient has had the premedication prescribed by the anaesthetist, but says that this need not matter as he has previously explained to her that unfortunately her illness may make more radical surgery necessary. There is, however, no indication that this has been done on either the existing consent form or the patient's records.

What do you do in these circumstances?

Study B5: A nurse/patient relationship?

A community psychiatric nurse visited a patient who had recently been discharged from hospital. She had spent a month in a psychiatric ward for treatment of her severe depression. When the nurse and the patient have been conversing for a while she (the patient) says that she is very worried about something, but not sure whether it would be right for her to talk to him (the nurse) about it.

Eventually the patient agrees to explain what it is that is so worrying her, but adds that she will not be prepared to talk to anyone else about it and is not prepared to make any kind of official complaint.

She then explains that the matter concerns a male member of the ward nursing staff who had cared for her while she was an inpatient. She says that she is not entirely clear about what happened, but she became particularly close to him and, she felt, he reciprocated those feelings. She adds that she is not sure how she feels about it now, but recalls that the particular nurse had offered to come and visit her after she had returned home and that she had replied that she did not want him to. She explains that she said this because the nurse also seemed very close to another woman patient and she did not want to come between them.

She reiterates that she does not wish to make any kind of complaint against the nurse who, she feels, means no harm. Indeed, she adds that, if she thought it might be acceptable and appropriate for her to see him again she would welcome that. In further explanation she adds that she and the nurse are the same age, and tells of a friend who, having first met him when she was in hospital with a broken leg, eventually married the doctor who had been caring for her at that time.

Were you this community psychiatric nurse, how would you respond to this new situation?

Study B6: The obstructive and abusive patient

Consider this situation. You are a community nursing sister in charge of a team of nurses. To one of them you have allocated the care of a man with leg ulcers. That care involves visiting the patient in his own home in order to change the dressings on his legs.

The nurse allocated to this patient's care finds that he experiences considerable pain when the dressings are changed, and he steadily becomes more and more difficult and obstructive. Initially he shouted abuse at the nurse and accused her of being thoroughly incompetent and unnecessarily rough. This then progresses to threatening to complain about her by writing to, or telephoning, his general practitioner to disclose how rough she was being. This then further progressed to him shouting the abuse very loudly and almost hysterically. This pattern of behaviour was relentless and upset the nurse to such a degree that, through negotiations with colleagues, she arranged to be accompanied by another member of the community nursing team whenever she called to change the dressings.

The patient's behaviour did not improve, despite the several nurses' attempts to discuss his problems with him in order to devise a means of allaying the discomfort he was apparently experiencing. In fact, it deteriorated further, even to the point of the patient picking up heavy ornaments and throwing them across the room. The spoken threats now included suggestions of violence towards the nurses who, by this stage, had become afraid to visit the patient, even in pairs.

Meanwhile the condition of the patient's leg ulcers was deteriorating and a number of nurses in the team were expressing reservations about whether they could ever cope with visiting this man again. The nurse to whom his treatment was allocated becomes concerned that she will be blamed for his deterioration and for not handling the admittedly difficult situation much better. She decides to place the whole picture before her team leader – the community nursing sister.

Faced with this difficult situation, what is she to do? It seems hardly reasonable to knowingly expose members of her team to the risk of physical harm? But there is still a patient in need of treatment.

Study B7: The manipulative teenager with anorexia

A 16-year-old girl has been admitted to a hospital ward because she is suffering from anorexia nervosa. She is a very intelligent child, being a year ahead at school and regarded as very gifted academically. She is articulate, but she is also manipulative.

She has come to an agreement with the medical team that she will allow herself to be fed by tube, indicating to them that she understands that if she is not assisted in this way she will die. That is the context of the dilemma. The dilemma itself arises when a nurse, working in the adjacent room, observes through a small gap in the curtains covering the dividing glass panels, that the girl patient, when she believes she is not observed, is detaching the feeding tube and wasting most of the feed into the sink.

The girl realises that she has been seen, and beckons the nurse to come into her room. The patient then explains to the nurse why she was running the liquid feed to waste. She says that she has been suffering with this illness for 3 years and no longer wants to cope with all the misery and pain. She says she is convinced that she will never get better and has lost the will to even try. She says that she wants relief at last from her suffering and wants to let herself die. She adds that she is now fully prepared for this to happen and, having made her decision, at last feels at peace with herself.

That said, she begs the nurse not to tell anyone else what she has observed or share the details of their conversation. She also states that, being 16 years of age and fully understanding the facts of her situation, she is legally in a position to take responsibility for her decision to accept or refuse treatment.

What is this nurse to do in this testing set of circumstances? Remember to consider the two key questions posed in this chapter's introductory text.

Study B8: Practice nurse – scope of role

Pleased with his success in obtaining a new post as a practice nurse with a large general medical practice, a nurse arrived at the practice premises for his first day. On arrival he found that it had been arranged for him to have a meeting early on that day with the practice manager. The practice manager was also still very new in post, having arrived only a few weeks previously. She had, until recently, been employed as the local branch manager for a major bank, but had felt like accepting a new challenge and believed that she could find it in this special aspect of health care management.

The new practice manager had been particularly keen to make a good impression, and to this end had been reading as much as she could find about various aspects of health care. One result of her reading was that she had noticed that a great deal had been written about the developing roles of nurses, and the ways in which some of them were accepting responsibility for a range of activities that had traditionally been regarded as solely within the medical practitioner's role. She was very keen for the practice to be seen as at the leading edge and wanted to increase the number of patients seen by the doctors by offloading some of their work.

To this end, when meeting the new nurse on his first morning, she handed to him a list of activities that she felt that he should undertake. The list included conducting a minor surgery clinic for the removal of 'lumps and bumps', running a well woman clinic, taking cervical smears and the total reorganisation of the arrangements for labelling and filing patients' records. Her justification for the latter item was that she looked to him to create a more confidential storage system – one which would limit the need for access to the records by people who were not themselves registered health professionals.

The nurse is asked to consider the list and discuss it with the practice manager a few days later. What might be the result of his consideration?

Study B9: Deleting previously-made records

To consider this study you must place yourself in the position of an agency nurse who, one day, presented herself to work on a hospital ward that was completely new territory for her. This was a ward that no longer used any handwritten nursing notes, a new computerised system having recently been introduced for all record-keeping purposes. No parallel written records were kept.

A registered nurse who was a permanent member of the ward staff introduced the new system to the agency nurse. She proudly opened the system and gained access to some records that she had made in relation to a particular patient the previous day. While this record was on the screen she (the ward nurse) observes two entries which she feels, in retrospect, are not entirely correct. Without hesitation, she deleted these entries and replaced them with other words and phrases, declaring that the system is very good and clever in that it allows this to be done, thus making it easy to make the records even more accurate.

The agency nurse is surprised by what she has seen, and recognises the inherent dangers of a system that allows not only the originator of the entry, but any person with access to the record to change it and leave no trace that this has been done. She mildly expresses her concern, but the ward nurse emphatically replies that it is an entirely acceptable practice.

In justification of action observed by the agency nurse she states that she had made the original record and she had demonstrated one of the advantages of the system. To this she added that, even with written records, the nurse would be entitled to tear up the notes that she had made if she subsequently considered them inaccurate and write a new version. Finally she told the agency nurse that if this worried her she could leave at the end of the shift and not return.

The agency nurse does not feel reassured by the justification she has heard. Would you? How does this system fit with your view of the purpose for which records are made? Once again, consider this study in the context of the two key questions in this chapter's introduction.

Study B10: A matter of standards

A nurse who had received her preregistration education and training in the United Kingdom and had current effective registration in that country had gone, under contract, to work in a hospital in a country in the Middle East.

Having settled into her new post, she became increasingly concerned about the generally poor standards of care. She was particularly concerned about the practice of one senior nurse whom she thought should be something of a role model for others but who was evidently seriously out of date with current good nursing practices and procedures.

Feeling so concerned, our nurse shared her thoughts and concerns with a nursing colleague who had been there longer. The response she received from that colleague was to agree with her conclusions and share her concern, but to add that, because they were working 'on foreign soil', there was no professional obligation for them to do anything about the situation. To that her colleague added that, were they to complain they had to recognise that they were in a country where they had no protection rights as employees and that the likely outcome would be that they would be sacked. This, she said, would not help the patients who were already suffering the effects of staff shortages.

Our nurse remains troubled. Is it the case that her professional obligations ceased as she left UK shores? She feels compromised by the situation in which she now finds herself.

Study B11: An issue of consent

In this study the setting is a surgical ward in a major hospital. A number of patients are to have their operations that morning, and one of the registered nurses is completing the required preparatory work. In the process, she notices that one of the patients does not appear to have signed a consent form. The patient confirms for her that this is correct.

The nurse attempts to contact the surgeon who is to perform the patient's operation, but a message is relayed back to her that he is already in the process of operating and that his junior doctor is assisting him. The message also conveys the request that the nurse obtain the consent on his behalf.

The operation which the patient is to have is apparently relatively minor. It involves the extraction of four wisdom teeth followed immediately by the removal of a small growth in the mouth. The patient is not to have any premedication and, apart from the absence of a signed consent form, is ready to go to the operating department.

The nurse now feels under pressure to obtain the consent in order that the patient can proceed to have the operation as planned without delay but, noting the specific wording of the consent form, remains anxious about doing so.

Is she worrying without cause, or is there a true dilemma here? How would you respond in this situation? Are there any 'What if?' questions you would want to consider?

Study B12: An offer of commercial sponsorship

A group of community midwives has decided that they wish to produce information on breast feeding for mothers in order to promote its benefits. It is intended also that the same text will provide practical advice on how to proceed when, breast-feeding having been established, the mother encounters difficulties. Their feeling is that, if only this information can be provided for mothers at an early stage and is supported by suitable printed material for easy reference, there will be an increase in the duration of time that many mothers will be able to continue breast-feeding. They intend that the booklet would also include details of a daytime 'help line' to the building at which they are based, the purpose of which would be to respond instantly to requests for information or advice.

While supporting the midwives in their desire to publish a booklet for this important purpose, their employer does not have funds available to pursue this venture. At this stage on to the scene with an offer to finance the venture steps a major manufacturer whose products include disposable nappies, other baby products and, most significantly in the context of this matter, baby foods. What they seek in return is to place advertising material within the booklet.

The time is soon to come when a representative of the company is to attend for a meeting to discuss the arrangements, so the midwives are endeavouring to prepare themselves and coordinate their views. At this stage some disagreement between them emerges.

On the one hand are those midwives who are willing to allow the company as much advertising space in the booklet as they request, feeling that if they do not take this stance they might never get the intended booklet published. They accept that there is something in the argument that the midwives, by distributing the booklet, might be seen as endorsing or recommending the company's products, but feel that the advantage to be gained outweighs that risk.

At the other extreme are those midwives who are extremely concerned about any connection being made between their names and this one company's products.

Can a balance be struck which does not compromise these midwives?

Study B13: A confidentiality test

A new patient has been admitted to a hospital ward following a car accident. He does not appear to have any major injuries, but has suffered concussion and is being kept in overnight for observation.

A nurse working the night shift is allocated the care of this patient. The patient has difficulty in sleeping, so, in response to his request, and her other duties allowing it, she spends some time in conversation with him. He had obviously found the experience of the accident unpleasant and disturbing, and was unsettled at now spending the night in strange surroundings. In the course of the conversation the patient begins to reveal some detailed information about himself to the nurse, including the fact that he has recently been diagnosed as HIV positive. He explains that he had not divulged this fact to anyone else, including those in the hospital who dealt with him at the time of admission, because he has not yet come to terms with this new knowledge about himself. He asks the nurse to respect his confidentiality and keep this information secret.

Once the patient has fallen asleep the nurse considers what, if anything, she should do with the information she now possesses. However, before she has come to any conclusion the patient's condition begins to deteriorate markedly. His level of consciousness reduces rapidly and he then suffers a cardiac arrest. The resuscitation team arrive in response to the nurse's call but their attempts to revive him are unfortunately not successful and he dies within a short time. The nurse has not, at this stage, revealed to anyone the information which the patient had shared with her in confidence. The patient's wife and two teenage children now arrive on the ward in response to the telephone call the nurse had made to them earlier.

The nurse is now asking herself two questions. Should she have revealed to other members of the hospital staff at an earlier stage the information she had been given? Now that the deceased man's wife has arrived, what should she now do with that information? She felt that she was in an extremely uncomfortable position as a result of the events of this night. How would you respond?

Study B14: A request for advocacy

Picture this scene. You are a health visitor whose practice base is a clinic building from which a general medical practice operates. One day, as you are walking along the clinic corridor, you encounter the teenage daughter of one of your current clients. The girl is obviously very distressed, so you take her aside into an available room, give her a drink and try to calm her down. The girl soon reveals to you the cause of her distress.

She tells you that she is pregnant and does not wish to have the baby, so for that reason has been to see her doctor to ask her to arrange an abortion. She adds that the doctor has agreed to do this, but, to her dismay, insists on informing the girl's parents about the consultation and decision. She says that the doctor has told her that, as she is only 15 years of age, she has no choice in the matter.

The girl begs the health visitor to help her and presses her to talk to the doctor. She explains that her parents are very religious and, if told about her predicament, will not only be devastated but will insist that she has the baby. She adds that she is desperately keen to maintain her good progress at school and is sure that, if she is compelled to have the baby, her career plans will suffer irredeemably.

The health visitor, who has a current professional connection with the family, agrees to talk to the doctor about the situation. Having accepted the request to intercede and be an advocate for this distressed girl, what arguments might she have to offer? What information can she offer the doctor? And what can she do if the doctor is not moved by her advocacy?

Study B15: An acceptable solution?

In the course of her work, a community nurse visits a physically and mentally handicapped adult who is being cared for by his parents at home. This man is desperate to be as independent as possible and the visit has been planned to consider how he might take more responsibility for his own prescribed medication as one way of responding to his wishes.

It emerges that, over a period of some years, he has needed to take a quantity of tablets and at various times of the day. He is not able to open the containers in which the medicines are supplied, but otherwise understands which tablets he needs to take and at which times, and explains this to the community nurse.

The parents explain exactly what their son is able to do in this respect. It appears that he is able to hold a cup, but does not have the manual dexterity to hold other and smaller objects. The parents also explain their proposed solution. This is that, at the start of each day, they put the prescribed tablets into three large cups for their son to take on his own at the appropriate times during the day. They add that they have done this on an experimental basis and it has worked well. They now wish the nurse's advice as to whether this can be regarded as an appropriate way to help their son in the future and enhance his feelings of independence.

What would you say to this request?

B16: Thoughtless redeployment

The combination of limited financial resources and increasing problems of recruitment of registered nurses has led a health authority to conduct a reappraisal of its policies for staffing at night.

One of the decisions made and announced is that, when the operating theatres are not in action during the night, the theatre nursing staff will be redeployed. The reaction of the theatre staff to this is not to be particularly worried, since in this large city general hospital the operating theatres are busy almost every night and, if they were allocated elsewhere, they would always be placed in support of other staff as the prospect would always exist of their recall to theatre if emergencies arose. They simply stated their expectation on this point to their managers and were told nothing to disillusion them.

Some weeks later, quite exceptionally, the operating theatre was not in action 3 hours into the night shift. The senior staff nurse on theatre duty was suddenly instructed to go to take charge of a large, busy paediatric ward in which there were a number of very ill children. She was told by the night sister that the unqualified staff on the ward would tell her about the patients as she did not have time to go to the ward herself.

Although she has been a registered nurse for 12 years, the theatre staff nurse has worked only in operating theatres for all of those 12 years. She has had no ward experience since registration and had only 8 weeks allocation to a paediatric ward when a student nurse.

What should this nurse do? She is aware of the expectation stated in the Code of Professional Conduct that she acknowledge the limits of her knowledge and competence. Will the children in the ward be better off with her or without her? Is there some other solution to offer? What would you have done in these circumstances?

Study B17: An explosive disclosure

In the course of private conversastion with an informal patient in a psychiatric unit a charge nurse was informed by that patient that, for a period of time in the recent past, he had sexually abused two young girls who were his nieces.

Concerned about the information he now possessed and being also concerned at the possibility of further such abuse directed to the same or other children, the charge nurse shared the information now in his possession with his immediate nurse manager.

His own professional superior told him that, as soon as such information began to emerge, he should have drawn the conversation to a close and withdrawn from the situation, since his own position might become compromised. The charge nurse, however, found that the situation was not as simple as that, since, with no indication of what might be to come, the patient suddenly blurted out the full facts. In any event, he was far from convinced about the validity of the advice he was being given which was to the effect that he should do nothing.

Clearly he will get no effective help or support from his manager and must make his own decision. What course of action would you recommend to him? Again, bear in mind the two questions posed in the opening section of this chapter.

Study B18: Avoiding stigma?

A nurse manager of a psychiatric unit was faced with a dilemma which was shared by some of the charge nurses within the unit of which he was the nurse manager.

The unit contained one 'secure' locked ward but also a number of wards which were not locked.

There were some patients on the unlocked wards whose condition and behaviour gave cause for serious concern. The psychiatrists, however, were reluctant to use their powers under the Mental Health Act to compulsorily detain these patients as they felt that to do so would 'stigmatise' them. These patients therefore remained in the unlocked wards where staffing levels and mix were geared to expectations of the anticipated type of occupants.

However, the same psychiatrists stated their requirement that the same patients, accommodated as informal patients in unlocked wards, must be 'specialled'. This they stated as meaning a one-to-one nurse/patient contact at all times, the nurse always to remain 'within arm's length' of the patient.

This nurse manager faces a testing dilemma. It not only challenges his professional authority and potentially strains the human resources he has to deploy beyond acceptable limits, but raises a serious matter of principle about patient treatment. Once again, consider the situation described in the light of the two standard questions posed in the chapter introduction.

Study B19: The wider public interest

A community psychiatric nurse found herself faced with a considerable dilemma relating to confidentiality arising out of her practice.

One of her clients was known by her to have been banned from driving following convictions for driving with a blood alcohol substantially above the limit and driving while uninsured. These offences and the resulting convictions had occurred before she became the nurse allocated to his case. As a result of her involvement she was also aware that he was receiving medication which might impair his judgment and make driving inadvisable.

She had felt for some time that she was developing a good and potentially therapeutic relationship with this client and had high hopes that it might succeed in achieving the breakthrough that a previous episode of inpatient treatment failed to achieve. The dilemma had arisen, however, because the nurse had now seen the client driving a car alone on a number of occasions in the busy town in which they both live.

What should the nurse do? On the one hand she recognises the risk of possible serious injury to her client or other people if he is involved in an accident because she has not informed the police. On the other hand she realises that if she does so inform, the therapeutic relationship which she believes to be developing with a chance of genuine progress will be shattered and any subsequent treatment programme rendered more difficult. She has quietly mentioned to him that she has seen him driving, but it has not achieved the change she hoped for.

Discuss, remembering the theoretical and practical questions set before you at the opening of this chapter.

Study B20: The personal and professional interface

A practice nurse employed by a large GP practice went home from work one day to find that her house had been broken into and possessions to the value of about £400 stolen. One of the missing items was a very unusual and distinctive bracelet of great sentimental value and a monetary value of some £400.

Three months later, when this nurse was on duty in the practice, a woman patient was directed to her room for some treatment. The nurse immediately noticed that the patient was wearing a bracelet exactly like that stolen from her home. The nurse was taken aback by this, but, with great self-control, said how very unusual the bracelet was and how much she admired it. The patient's response was to say 'Yes, it is lovely isn't it. I was given it as a present about 12 weeks ago'. There was no suggestion of guilt or anxiety in this response.

The nurse's suspicions were aroused by this response. What should she do? Her financial loss is being met by her insurers, but she naturally feels aggrieved by the invasion of her home and the theft. On the one hand, the woman may have been given the bracelet by someone who had purchased it through proper channels. On the other hand, to go to the police may lead to those responsible for this and other burglaries. It is clear that the police could do nothing if she does not disclose the patient's name and address, but that would be a breach of confidentiality. Could she justify that action? Remember the two core questions as you consider this unusual situation in which one registered nurse found herself.

Appendix 1

Decisions and/or Discussion of the Professional Conduct Committee Case Studies in Chapter 13 and the Accountability/Ethical Dilemma Case Studies in Chapter 14

Introduction

The reader should not necessarily approach these pages in the expectation of finding what is, without any doubt or reservation, the one definitive right answer. Things are not as simple as that.

In respect of the 'A' case studies based on UKCC Professional Conduct Committee cases, the following text informs you what the Committee decided on the day. The decision is the result of the individual judgment of the members being drawn together to arrive at a corporate conclusion. There is no one right answer to any of the cases.

Similarly, in respect of the 'B' studies, do not approach the following text looking for definitive answers to the various professional dilemmas described. The brief commentary provided in respect of each of them is offered only as a basis for further consideration and discussion. Professional practice necessarily involves the individual in considering a situation, exercising her or his judgment in that situation and being able to justify the decision made and consequent action.

Case A1: Decision

Having considered the evidence in its context, the Committee determined that the proven charge relating to leaving the home without a registered nurse should not be regarded as misconduct, since it was exceptional, accidental and of very short duration. It found all the other proven charges to be misconduct in a professional sense. The respondent's lawyer submitted in evidence a number of testimonials from former residents of the home and relatives of residents.

The Committee decided to remove the respondent's name from the professional register.

Case A2: Decision

The Committee decided that all the proven charges against each of the two respondents did amount to misconduct in a professional sense. Since both respondents had declined to attend the hearing and had not submitted any written evidence in mitigation which could be considered prior to the final decisions being made, there was nothing further available to assist the Committee. The Committee was advised, however, that both respondents had been dismissed by their employer as a result of these matters, that both had appealed against that decision, that respondent A's appeal had been rejected but that respondent B's appeal had been upheld. In her case, dismissal was replaced with demotion and a requirement to work under supervision for 1 year. Respondent B did not return, however, being on certificated sick leave for some months before retiring on grounds of ill health.

The Committee decided to remove respondent A's name from the register. In respect of respondent B, it decided to administer a formal caution which would remain on her record for 5 years and be made evident to any potential employer seeking confirmation of her registration status.

Case A3: Decision

The Committee, after due deliberation, found the facts alleged in the charge to be proved to the required standard. Had the respondent chosen to attend, it would have been open to her, either directly or through a representative, to argue that the proven facts, when considered in their context rather than in isolation, did not amount to professional misconduct. Without the benefit of hearing any such representations, the Committee decided that misconduct had been proved.

At the next stage, the Committee received a letter addressed to it from the respondent and a quantity of references. After further deliberation in camera, the Committee announced its decision to administer a formal caution which would remain on file for 5 years and would be taken into account should the respondent be found guilty of any further misconduct within that period. The Chairman emphasised that the decision must not be taken as condoning or excusing the respondent's actions and omissions in any way.

Case A4: Decision

The Committee had little hesitation in deciding that the facts did amount to misconduct in a professional sense. Had the respondent attended, she could at this stage, either directly or through a representative, have submitted evidence or argument in mitigation. In the absence of any such evidence the Committee heard from a senior nursing manager of the hospital at which the respondent had been employed.

This provided a description of a person who, since her original registration as a nurse 18 years earlier, had a career with no evident blemish. In addition to the acquisition of additional academic and professional qualifications, she had won a number of prestigious awards and scholarships, had contributed to a variety of books and journals through her own writings and book reviews, was a Supervisor of Midwives and an examiner for midwives taking higher diplomas and degrees.

She had been with the same employing authority for a number of years, having been Head of the Midwifery Training School before moving to her final managerial post. She resigned that post following her court appearance. The witness was not aware if she had obtained further employment.

The Committee decided to remove this respondent's name from the register with immediate effect.

Case A5: Decision

The Committee decided to reject the application. In doing so it advised the applicant to contact the Nurses Welfare Service to seek advice about planning for the future.

Case A6: Decision

The members of the Committee were concerned to note that the respondent's considerable sickness absence over a substantial period had not been noted by her managers sufficiently for her to be referred to the hospital's Occupational Health Department. Similar concern was felt about the frailties of the financial system which allowed the offences to be committed. They were not, however, convinced by the arguments submitted in mitigation, noting particularly that, although they had been told that the offences were 'isolated and uncharacteristic', they had been perpetrated over a period of several weeks. The Committee therefore decided to remove the respondent's name from the register with immediate effect.

Case A7: Decision

The members of the Committee decided that removal from the register was necessary in this case, even recognising its limitations in respect of residential home posts.

Case A8: Decision

Without the opportunity to question this nurse and form a view of her awareness of her professional responsibilities, but mindful of the fact that she had betrayed the trust of a vulnerable elderly person, the Committee decided to remove her name from the register with immediate effect.

Case A9: Decision

In announcing the Committee's decision the Chairman told the respondent nurse that to be found guilty of professional misconduct by the regulatory body's Professional Conduct Committee in a public hearing was a very serious matter. However, noting and taking account of the evidence it had heard about her performance in her new employment, having formed a view of her retrospective assessment of her own conduct and having studied the supportive testimonials it had received, the Committee had decided not to remove this nurse's name from the register.

It had decided instead to issue a formal caution which would remain on record for 5 years and would be made known to any person seeking confirmation of her registration status. It would also be brought forward as history of previous misconduct if, within that five-year period, any further misconduct was proved against her by a successor committee. The chairman stated the expectation that the nurse would now study the Code of Professional Conduct and apply the standards which it describes and promotes, in her future practice.

Case A10: Decision

The Committee's Chairman told the respondent that, had the hearing taken place shortly after the convictions for the offences listed in the charges, it was almost certain that he would have been removed from the register. However, because of the lapse in time since those events, he had been able to take steps, clearly successfully, to rehabilitate himself, as the excellent reports and references had confirmed for the Committee. The members were pleased that, from the time he began to seek employment, he had hidden nothing from any potential employer, so there had been no risk of an employer taking him on while unaware of the background.

In these circumstances, the Committee decided that, although his actions were undoubtedly serious and were undoubtedly misconduct in a professional sense, he should be given a formal caution and his name should not be removed from the register.

The fact that the formal caution and the reasons for it would be made known to any person seeking confirmation of his registration status was explained, as was the fact that this situation applied for a five-year period.

Case A11: Decision

Quite clearly the members of the Committee would have preferred to make their decision after having the opportunity to meet and question the respondent. Since she had not provided them with this opportunity, the Professional Conduct Committee resolved to remove her name from the register and, in notifying her of the decision in writing, to advise her of the procedures to be followed if, at some future date, she decided to make an application for restoration.

Case A12: Decision

Not surprisingly, the Committee was concerned at the evident deficiencies in the practice environment at the time, not least in respect of its arrangements to ensure the competence of its professional staff and for the maintenance of important equipment. Even making allowances for that, its members took the view that this respondent midwife had failed in a significant way and was not convinced by her representative's statements on her behalf. The decision was to remove her name from the professional register.

Case A13: Decision

The decision of the Professional Conduct Committee was to remove this nurse from the professional register. As is normal in these circumstances, that decision was confirmed to her in writing, together with information about the procedures to be followed should she, at some future stage, apply for restoration.

Case A14: Decision

Decisions in cases of this kind are always difficult. They are difficult because of the known tendency of many former alcohol-dependent people to break down in spite of their stated resolve. They are also difficult because you know that nursing is a profession which involves a considerable amount of stress. In many respects the decision whether or not to restore is a bigger one than whether or not to remove from the register.

In this case the Committee, having had the opportunity to meet and question the applicant, this being supplemented by access to some helpful reports and references, decided to accept his application. He was, of course, told that his previous removal would, within the following 5 years, be made known to any person wishing to confirm his registration status. A strong caution as to his future conduct was expressed.

Case A15: Decision

Indicating that its decision should not be seen as condoning or excusing his past actions, the Committee decided to administer a formal caution as to his future conduct, the conditions described in other cases again applying.

Case A16: Decision

The respondent in this case was in serious contravention of the Introduction and clauses 1 and 9 of the Code of Professional Conduct. She had seriously abused her privileged access to the homes and property of an extremely vulnerable client group.

The manner in which she stepped in and out of her professional role, going as a friend to help pack but changing back to 'the nurse' to write misleading notes about the alleged confused state of the patients was regarded by the Committee as particularly nasty and devious. The patients went to different places at different times so the risk of one patient's concern about her linking up with other such concerns was remote.

In spite of the fact that the respondent was said to be skilful and competent and that she formed good relationships with patients and their relatives the Committee felt that the public interest required that she be removed from the register and so ordered.

Case A17: Decision

You were probably tempted to regard this case as fictional. Unfortunately it states things as they happened in this psychiatric unit.

Quite apart from the behaviour of the respondent in the case, there is cause for concern about the limited attention given to this patient during the morning shift, and the inadequacy of the hand-over report that left the respondent inadequately informed when first encountering the patient.

None of that, however, justified his reactions to the patient's request. There were other staff on duty and it was never argued in the respondent's defence that the unit was short of staff at the time.

The Committee decided to remove this nurse from the register and also to send a transcript of the hearing to the Chairman of the health authority as a means of drawing its concerns about the management of the unit to his attention.

Case A18: Decision

The Committee retired for a long time to discuss the case, that fact alone being indicative of the seriousness with which they regarded the offences. In announcing the decision the Chairman of the Committee made that point, and further indicated that they had not been impressed by the allegations made in the course of the defence against the respondent's professional colleagues, claiming that they had behaved inappropriately and acted with something less than professional competence, since such allegations had not in any way been substantiated. The Chairman added that, since on the respondent's instructions her barrister had contested the facts of the case for two days, it was impossible for the Committee to see it (as had been urged upon them) as 'merely an admitted error'.

On behalf of the Committee the Chairman indicated that, even had the situation contained factors that got in the way of delivery of safe care, it expected someone of the educational and professional background concerned to be challenging of such adverse situations and not accepting of them. In the event the Chairman told the respondent that the Committee had been divided on the matter and that the respondent had come extremely close to removal from the register, but that on balance it had been decided not to take that decision but to speak words of caution and counsel. The Chairman emphasised very strongly that the decision not to remove the respondent from the register in no way condoned her conduct in respect of the patient who was placed at risk by her actions.

Case A19: Decision

The Chairman indicated, in giving the Committee's judgment, that to keep and maintain adequate records was both a fundamental feature of health visiting practice and of professional accountability. She added that clause 2 of the UKCC Code of Professional Conduct makes an omission to do something for which you have responsibility just as serious as an act of commission.

However, noting the numerous testimonials concerning her personal and professional qualities, her obvious commitment and innovative practice, and the climate of change and disagreement in which she had been working, the Committee decided to take no further action on the misconduct proved against her.

It was noted that she had acknowledged her own shortcomings in record-keeping and recognised that she must personally address the issue if she returned to health visiting practice which she was legally able to do.

Case A20: Discussion

The text of this case study drew attention to the positive steps taken by the responsible professional manager in respect of the three respondents. It also drew attention to the various points made in mitigation on their behalf and to the concerns which the proven facts had raised in the minds of the Committee.

Before announcing the decision the Chairman stated that the impression to emerge from the case had been that of a conspiracy of silence which was only broken as a result of action taken by newly qualified nurses. This the Committee regarded as courageous, demonstrating their awareness of their professional responsibility as stated in the UKCC's Code of Professional Conduct. The Committee particularly praised the steadfastness of purpose of one witness who, from the time she observed things which caused her grave concern when she was a student, had persisted in her determination to bring those concerns into the open and achieve proper investigation of them in spite of the obstruction she encountered.

After considerable deliberation, and putting in the balance the reprehensible actions or omissions of the three respondents, the things which emerged about them in mitigation, and the subsequent extremely positive enabling work done by their senior manager following his decision not to dismiss them from employment, the Committee decided that no further action should be taken in any of the three cases other than to give some advice as to the respondents' future conduct.

The Chairman, however, reiterated that the misconduct of which the enrolled nurse had been found guilty was grave since she had handled patients inappropriately, abrogated her responsibility of care, and failed to accord respect to the beliefs of a patient, in all of which respects she had contravened the UKCC's expectations of practitioners as set out in the Code of Professional Conduct. As for the ward sister, it was emphasised that a person holding such a post has a responsibility to ensure that the standards of practice on a ward are acceptable, that activities are monitored, and that complaints are appropriately investigated irrespective of the views held about a member of staff about whom complaints were received. In respect of the nurse manager, the Chairman indicated the Committee's view that she was a victim of circumstances who had acted inappropriately when placed in an impossible position by her manager.

Case A21: Decision

The Professional Conduct Committee which heard this case, like its equivalent on many other days, was almost certainly ready to forgive a genuine mistake made under pressure at the end of a busy day. What it could not forgive was the dishonesty with which the mistake was compounded when the matter of the missing instrument came to light.

It seemed to be a case in which pride got in the way of taking an action in the patient's interests.

It should be noted from the text of the case study that, by the time of the hearing, the respondent had obtained a post as a theatre sister, this seemingly being obtained without references being taken up, such a high premium being placed on operating theatre skills.

After very careful consideration the Committee decided to postpone judgment for 3 months (the shortest possible period of postponement) and to require for the resumed hearing a reference from the respondent's new employer which had to be written with knowledge of the facts.

Although it is fairly incidental to this case as it affected the respondent, it is worth recording that the Committee felt that the response of the two night nurses had been less than adequate, although the degree of response from them was probably fairly typical of that which might have been expected from the average registered nurse.

Case A22: Decision

It is obviously preferable for a newly registered nurse to obtain her first experience as a staff nurse on familiar territory. Where this does not prove possible, and particularly where the search for work results in a young person moving a long distance to an unfamiliar setting, it is incumbent on those who employ her to ensure that their introduction to the place and their induction to the work is thorough and comprehensive.

The Committee members were extremely concerned that, in this case, such did not appear to have happened, since as the induction programme was of only 3 days duration, it gave very little opportunity for a thorough orientation to a different setting. In addition, it became clear that, since this respondent was a RSCN and the night sisters were not, she (though newly registered) was led to believe that they regarded her as the expert on paediatrics and there was not a great deal of point in calling upon the night sisters. The Committee members were also concerned at the fact that those who employed her seemed to be expecting her to demonstrate the same degree of knowledge, skill and maturity as they reasonably could from a person of several years standing on the register.

The facts were clearly set out in the case study, and it is indicated that they were admitted. The young woman who appeared with an excellent solicitor did not in any way wish to argue that those facts were not misconduct, and the Committee so found.

At the mitigation stage it emerged that, unlike many others, she had busily occupied her time with further education at a polytechnic to obtain a professional qualification in social work so that, were her registration as a nurse removed, (and she was emphatic that she did not wish that it happen), she was equipped to work in another professional sphere. The Committee respected her greatly for these endeavours, and noted the excellent references she had received in respect of work in an unqualified capacity that she had been doing in both health and social work settings to help fund her further studies.

The members felt that this respondent was very much a victim of the circumstances in which she worked, were satisfied that she had learnt a great deal and grown in insight as a result of her unfortunate experience, and decided that a few words of caution and counsel was quite sufficient.

Case A23: Decision

This was an example of a nurse who was taking advantage of her position and clearly contravening clauses 1 and 9 of the Council's Code of Professional Conduct.

Had the matter not come to light the respondent would have obtained for £140 an antique dining table which would comfortably seat eight, with a set of eight matching antique chairs, and a number of other valuable items which together were of far greater value. Although the patient might have been unusual in respect of those who are the subject of Court of Protection Orders, in that she was still regarded as able to live alone, she was certainly deemed incapable of managing her own financial affairs and it was in this respect that particular advantage was taken of her.

The Committee also particularly disliked the way in which the young community service volunteer, newly moved away from home because of the difficulty of finding work in his own locality, was used first as a means of moving the furniture and of handing over the money, and subsequently that attempts were made to get him to say that the money was a loan from the respondent so that he could buy furniture for his deprived parents. The respondent said that they were apparently in serious need, without carpets and bedding and the like, so an antique table and chairs would not have seemed the thing that they most urgently required.

The decision of the Committee was to remove this lady from the register.

Case A24: Decision

As in a substantial percentage of the cases heard by the Committee, the respondent in this case was not the only person with something to answer for. Indeed, it could be argued that she was something of a scapegoat since she was not the senior of the three nurses on duty at the time, and although she was the one who had turned the alarm on the machine off, one of her colleagues had subsequently undertaken the patient's observations and had not turned it on again, and in any event the practice of so doing was well established and engaged in by medical and nursing staff. It rather seemed as if, since a patient had died, the health authority had to have a sacrificial lamb, so this nurse was dismissed from employment and made the subject of allegations of misconduct to the statutory body.

The Committee felt that her actions had been less than satisfactory, but also felt that others not before them and who had not been made the subject of any complaint were as culpable or possibly more culpable.

Given the culpability of others and the previously good record of this nurse who was clearly the wiser for the experience, the Committee, although finding her guilty of misconduct, decided that no further action was needed other than that she be given some words of caution and counsel.

Study B1: Discussion

The difficulty with which the department sister is faced is that, although she has a duty of confidentiality to the patient, she will also feel some obligation to assist the police with their inquiries into a very serious assault. To assist nurses on its register, the regulatory body in the United Kingdom (the UKCC) has provided guidance on the nurse's duty of confidentiality in the booklet *Guidelines for Professional Practice*. This document, at paragraph 27, specifically refers to problems in Accident and Emergency Departments involving the police and advise that, if a decision is made to release confidential information, the person taking that decision must be able to justify it as an action to serve the wider public interest. The department sister may conclude that the wider public interest will be best served by providing information to the police because it will help to bring the perpetrator of the assault to justice. She will also be mindful of the current fearful state of the patient's relatives.

It might, of course, be the case that, unless the patient, once sufficiently recovered, is willing to identify his attacker and assist the police as they prepare a prosecution, any information given by the department sister to the police at this early stage will have no ultimate benefit. This might lead her to state that she cannot divulge the information the police are seeking at this stage, but that she will contact them as soon as the patient is able and willing to respond to their questions.

In respect of the police officers' request to speak to the patient's relatives, this must be seen as a decision for them. The department sister could certainly ask the question and, assuming an affirmative answer, provide a suitable confidential setting for an interview.

Study B2: Discussion

Situations of this kind are particularly difficult to manage. The nurse will want to respect the resident's privacy, but at the same time will want to protect her from the harm that she may suffer if she wanders into potential danger again. It is to be expected that she will be aware of her legal and professional duty to protect this lady. The UKCC document (referred to in respect of B1) comments on the extent of this duty.

The care plan for the resident must be prepared with due attention to the circumstances. Would it be appropriate for the resident to be constantly accompanied by a staff member, always assuming this was possible? Alternatively, is a check made by a specific staff member at regular intervals likely to serve the purpose and be more manageable? Neither of these approaches can be adopted if the staff complement does not allow, and it is quite possible that they are not economically feasible in a residential home of this kind. There are very practical questions for the nurse to consider.

It will also be necessary for her to consider the cause of the problem. Nursing expertise in the care of the elderly will undoubtedly be of benefit at this stage. Discussion with other staff members is obviously important. It might emerge from this that assistance be sought from other professional disciplines including, for example, a psychiatrist specialising in the mental health of elderly persons, or a community psychiatric nurse. It may emerge that this residential home setting is no longer appropriate for this resident and it would, in those circumstances, be wrong of the staff to keep her there for commercial reasons.

It has to be recognised that (in the United Kingdom), unless the resident is so mentally ill that she can be detained in a suitable place under the Mental Health Act, it is extremely difficult to prevent her from wandering. How important it therefore becomes that the team caring for this resident (and others) can be seen to be well organised and coordinated, and that its members maintain records that demonstrate that the standard of care provided was appropriate and the duty of care observed in all respects.

Study B3: Discussion

This is a serious dilemma for the charge nurse. In the United Kingdom he will certainly need to take account of the Code of Professional Conduct, one clause within which requires that, as an aspect of his accountability, he 'refuse any gift, favour or hospitality from patients or clients in your care which might be interpreted as seeking to exert influence to obtain preferential consideration'.

Is the patient trying to obtain preferential consideration? Is she using this as a means of expressing guilt for her past demands? Or is she simply grateful for the service provided for her by the charge nurse? If he seeks to dissuade her this may cause her great distress. If he does not, and subsequently does benefit, other staff might be critical of him and suggest that he often deferred to the patient's wishes in the expectation of reward. It would certainly have made life easier for him if the patient had made no such declaration. Since she has, it might be wise to persuade the patient to explain her intentions directly to a more senior member of the hospital staff in the absence of the charge nurse. Are there really no relatives who might emerge to challenge a will couched in these terms?

In the end, nothing can stop the patient making her will in this way if she chooses, but the charge nurse concerned should do his best to ensure that it does not appear to anyone that any of his actions were directed to achieve this outcome.

Study B4: Discussion

Many ethical dilemmas in professional practice concern the often difficult issue of consent. A section of the UKCC guidelines (referred to earlier) addresses the subject, and there is a considerable amount of other published material to assist the reader to consider the subject – particularly its legal aspects – in some depth. A nurse who has given the subject some consideration in general terms is better placed to make an appropriate decision when suddenly faced with a problematic set of circumstances, as was the nurse in this study.

The difficulty arises in this situation from the fact that the patient has been given a premedication of a powerful drug. The 'relaxed feeling' she describes appears to suggest that it has already exerted its influence. Is she, therefore, able to appreciate the significance of any new information put to her as a prelude to seeking her putting her signature to a new consent form authorising more radical surgery with one certain outcome? Might it not be best for the surgery to be deferred and for her to return to the ward pending her being able to give consent which is truly informed?

There might, however, be some potential danger for the patient in the surgical operation being even slightly delayed. This appears to be the surgeon's position. Only he knows the details of his earlier conversation with the patient, but it had culminated in the completion of the existing consent form, so how much reliance can be placed on his assertion that he has explained to the patient that more radical surgery might be necessary? There might be some possible merit in seeking a view from the patient's husband, since the patient might have reported her discussion with the surgeon to him in considerable detail. He, however, cannot give a lawful consent on behalf of the patient.

Study B5: Decision

It is, of course, a fact that many practitioners in the health care field first met their eventual partner in a professional capacity. It is important to recognise, however, that, as a general rule, developing a relationship with a patient is to be avoided. This is particularly the case where the setting in which practitioner and patient meet is concerned with the treatment of mental illness. In these situations there is the potential for the practitioner – nurse, doctor, etc. – to drift into a form of contact which can become an abuse of their professional position. The UKCC has provided no very specific guidance on this point, but the Code of Professional Conduct does require that nurses avoid any abuse of their privileged relationship with patients.

The circumstances described in this study raise a number of issues for the nurse involved to consider. First, he has his professional relationship with the patient to safeguard. If he decides to tell an appropriate person at the hospital what the patient has told him when he does not have her consent, her trust in him will have gone. He will recognise, however, that, if the patient's perception of events in the hospital is accurate, other patients may be exposed to inappropriate advances from the hospital nurse concerned. He is also aware that, if his patient is not willing to make an official complaint, no action is possible.

He will need to consider whether what he is hearing from the patient may be fabrication rather than truth, bearing in mind the vulnerable state in which she had been that led to her hospital admission. Taking time to explore with the patient her recollection of events might assist, as also might the involvement of a nursing or medical professional colleague. It is not an easy situation. Hopefully the patient might help to resolve it, but if not it possibly pits losing her trust against protecting other patients.

Study B6: Discussion

The situation described is an extremely difficult one for any nurse, no matter how experienced they may be. Clearly no professional nurse would ever wish to withdraw from providing care for a patient, and there can only be very limited circumstances in which this could be seen as necessary and therefore acceptable. The sections of the UKCC 'Guidelines' document on both duty of care and consent offer some insights that are relevant to this difficult situation.

The study focuses attention on the problem from the perspective of the Team Leader to whom the nurse directly involved has taken the problem. In her approach to the situation she has a duty to the patient, but a duty also to the members of her nursing team.

It would seem wise for her to personally experience the difficulty described to her by accompanying the nurse involved on her next visit to treat the patient. Assuming the patient is unmoved by her requests for cooperation and improvement, she might choose to involve his general medical practitioner who might consider whether the patient's current medication is appropriate and possibly consider whether some other specialist medical or nursing help is necessary. You might have other options to suggest.

Whatever decision is made, it must then be kept under review and the members of the nursing team must feel understood and supported by their managers.

Study B7: Discussion

This nurse has a major problem to deal with. It is to be hoped that she is a person who reads quality newspapers and professional journals and, as a result, has some awareness of the issues that surround anorexia.

This study is basically about consent, so access to the guidance on that subject is important. One of the major points to arise here is that of 'capacity'. Even though the individual patient concerned is right to assert that she is now of an age to lawfully give or withhold consent to treatment, this does not necessarily mean that, at this point in time, she has the mental capacity or competence to exercise that right. In cases such as this it is often deemed necessary to seek an 'Order' from the Courts to authorise treatment.

There is material in this case for lengthy discussion, as there is for varying opinions about the course of action to be pursued. It would seem unwise for this nurse to seek to resolve it without recourse to at least one other professional opinion, in spite of the girl's clear request. This is particularly important, bearing in mind that the Courts have become involved in reasonably similar cases. This may well be one of those occasions when the patient has unreasonable expectations of the professional practitioner concerned. It is important that professional practitioners, whoever they may be, have the capacity to recognise when a situation with which they are faced is beyond their experience and the humility to ask for another opinion. There is no one answer, and no easy answer in the circumstances described.

Study B8: Discussion

The scope of nursing practice has been the subject of considerable debate for some time past, and this remains the situation at the time of writing of this book. The UKCC has published its position and guidance on the subject in its booklet *The Scope of Professional Practice* which has its source in the Code of Professional Conduct. Invitations to develop the scope of your practice can be flattering and interesting. It is important, however, to consider whether such developments can be accommodated without neglecting other core aspects of your role that cannot be delegated. It is also essential that, before drawing into his practice some new activity, the nurse is quite sure of his knowledge and skill to perform it safely and to a good standard.

This study provides an example of the nurse being pulled in two directions at once. He is being expected to take on some of what has been traditionally regarded as the doctor's work (though there is no law in the United Kingdom that imposes that limit), but at the same time is expected to take on an administrative function that might be a waste of professional time that can be better used. In respect of the record system, perhaps he needs diplomatically to help the manager to understand the essential elements of a confidential system, together with the need for clear rules about non-disclosure that apply to all staff, and to make himself available to assist in the development of appropriate policies and practices.

Study B9: Discussion

The fact that the agency nurse has no desire to work on this ward again does not negate the fact that she bears a legal and professional duty to practise to an acceptable standard. What she is faced with is not in accord with that duty. If she has familiarised herself with the UKCC's 'Standards for Records and Record Keeping' she will be aware of this. The basic principles that apply to record-keeping should not disappear simply because a computerised system is in use.

The system in use here puts at risk the ability of the staff to provide continuity of care with confidence and, incidentally, endangers staff who, if the subject of complaint, will become unable to demonstrate that their care of a patient has been appropriate and their duty of care fulfilled if the record has been deleted. The agency nurse would seem entitled to report her concerns to a more senior person, given the requirement of the Code of Professional Conduct that she do so when 'safe and appropriate care for patients cannot be provided'.

Study B10: Discussion

What a difficult situation for the nurse. The fact that she is working outside the United Kingdom does not negate her UK registration. The expectations that her regulatory body has of her (stated in the Code of Professional Conduct) therefore continue to apply. Clauses 11, 12 and 13 of that code have a particular relevance in this situation, focusing attention as they do on the duty of care which she bears.

This study is concerned with what has come to be described colloquially as 'whistleblowing'. Seeking an opinion from a colleague and seeking to join them with you in making representations can often help. In this situation she has already done that and, while finding agreement with her description of the problem, has found no support. Indeed, the suggestion is that to take any action would only worsen the situation for the patients. Is there any action you think she might take, other than to leave so as not to feel tarnished and compromised? This is a most unenviable position.

Study B11: Discussion

Although this study is about consent, it does not have the complexities that were a feature of B4. The UKCC's guidance emphasises the importance of the person who is to perform a procedure being the person who should obtain the consent, while allowing that there may be some emergency situations in which this might be done by another professional practitioner.

It is difficult to categorise this case as an emergency, yet it might seem petty for the nurse not to do as requested. It is evident that this is not one of those settings in which there is a protocol in place against which it is selected nurses who routinely provide information to and obtain consent from patients.

The nurse needs to consider the principles that are relevant to the situation. Has the patient enough information to make an informed decision? If not, does the nurse possess the knowledge to provide that information, including a description of any possibly significant risks? Should something go awry, the possibility of some comeback on the nurse for not explaining a specific risk that has now materialised cannot be ruled out, but the prospect of this happening is remote. It is, perhaps, appropriate for the nurse to proceed as requested if she can answer with an unequivocal 'Yes' to the latter question. It would certainly seem essential, if the nurse takes this action, that it be a matter of record that she has done so.

Study B12: Discussion

Health care professionals in the United Kingdom increasingly find themselves operating in an environment in which commercial factors introduce the risk of their independent judgement appearing to be compromised. Both the Code of Professional Conduct and the UKCC Guidelines that flow from it indicate the basic principles that a nurse, midwife or health visitor should apply in this kind of situation. The fact remains, however, that in situations such as this, what is acceptable and what unacceptable is often a matter of subjective judgment.

Is it likely that the new mothers who receive the booklet will leap to the conclusion that, by handing it to them the midwives are overtly endorsing the particular company's products? Is there any prospect that the presence of the advertisement will, even in some subliminal way, undermine the message of the text of the booklet? Is it not the case that many publications do contain advertisements that largely go ignored?

The company's motives are unlikely to be entirely altruistic, but it might be content with the good will that it receives for its sponsorship. It might well accept the insertion of a brief declaration that the fact that the midwives provide the booklets to the mothers does not necessarily mean that they endorse the company's products. Alternatively it might be persuaded to offer sponsorship simply in return for a 'sponsored by...' acknowledgement. These alternatives appear to offer the benefit of achieving publication without compromise to the individual practitioners, yet still allowing the company to make an appropriate connection between itself and the profession of midwifery. There may be other options that you can identify.

Study B13: Discussion

This is another profoundly difficult situation. The nurse's duty of confidentiality to the patient (something that does not die with the death of a patient) has come into direct conflict with another duty – that to the man's wife. It might be that, without knowing it, his wife (and just possibly his children) have become infected.

Whatever her decision, she needs to be able to justify it to herself and, if there are any repercussions, to others. Is this really something that she can avoid sharing with at least one fellow health professional and joining them in the decision-making process? It seems an excessive burden to bear alone at a time when so much care is delivered by teams of mixed professional background.

The UKCC and various professional bodies have published documents providing information about AIDS and HIV. There are a number of impressive charities in the AIDS field from whom advice might be sought on a confidential and fairly hypothetical basis. In the end, however, the nurse has to make a decision. What have you decided to do? If you decide to disclose information to the man's newly bereaved wife, how is it to be done?

Study B14: Discussion

In the United Kingdom a young person under the age of 16 years can consent to treatment provided that they have a sufficient understanding of their condition and the treatment proposed. Any health professional endeavouring to come to a decision in a case such as that described has to form a view as to whether that level of understanding exists in a particular case. Presumably the doctor believes that it does, since he appears to have agreed to her request. It is the best interests of the young person that are to be regarded as paramount.

It might prove that, as a result of her discussion with the doctor, they come to an agreement about the appropriate course of action and that it is not to inform the parents. If that is not the result the health visitor is faced with a difficult situation. There is nothing she can do to prevent the medical practitioner from informing the parents of the situation and his intention to arrange a termination. She might possibly press for the passing of information to the parents to be delayed pending a discussion within the practice professional team, thus taking a wider range of views into account. That course of action might at least have the merit of avoiding continuing conflict within the professional team. You may have other options to propose. It is not an easy situation, that is certain.

Study B15: Discussion

It is to be hoped that the nurse, if practising in the United Kingdom, is familiar with the UKCC's publication *Standards for the Administration of Medicines*. On the face of it, the parents' plan would appear to be at odds with what that document advocates as best practice. Recognising that, the nurse must look at the specific circumstances of the person and the domestic context in which the medicines have to be administered.

It is evident that this young handicapped adult is striving for maximum independence within his limitations, and that his parents, quite properly, wish to foster that ambition. His best interests, in this setting, would appear to justify something very different from what would be acceptable in hospital practice.

This study serves as a useful reminder that, although official advice and guidance is important, professional practitioners must often make decisions as to the best course of action to follow in circumstances which do not match the ideal. That is what professional judgment is about.

Study B16: Discussion

The events really began when the staff were told of the redeployment plan, but did not ask for confirmation in writing of their assumption, or alternatively for instruction to render them competent for any wards to which they might be directed.

As a first move the nurse refused to go, stating to the night sister that it would be dangerous. She cited in aid clause 4 of the Code of Professional Conduct and was unimpressed by the night sister telling her she must go as there was nobody else to go. The night sister called the night nurse manager to speak to the nurse. She repeated the demand, but supplemented it with some emotional blackmail statements about the poor children in danger. Initially the nurse asked why one of the night sisters was not covering the ward in that case, and repeated her refusal.

After further pressure from her two superiors she said that she would go to the ward, but only after she had sat and written a document stating all the reasons why she felt it to be wrong. She said she would give one copy to the nurse manager, send one to the general manager and keep the third herself for a long time in case there were any long-term repercussions of the events of the night. Then she went. Three hours later there was a rush of emergency admissions and the nurse was recalled to the operating department.

Study B17: Discussion

The nurse in this case was justifiably disturbed by the response and attitude of his immediate manager. He convinced himself that he could not limit his concern to the one person who was his patient at the time but must have concern also for other vulnerable young people who would be in contact with this patient when he was discharged in the near future.

Given his belief that the patient was telling the truth and genuinely wanted to make known his past behaviour in this request, in spite of his manager's comments (which, surprisingly were supported by the psychiatrist), the nurse shared his information with the psychiatric social worker and together they initiated some appropriate action.

Study B18: Discussion

The contention of the nurse manager is that to do what the psychiatrists want would be tantamount to unlawful seclusion. It would certainly be an infringement of the freedom of the individual patients concerned. In addition, to comply with the stated requirement was not possible with the staffing levels existing and to even try would greatly reduce the service available to the other patients. In this he was supported by the charge nurses.

He therefore insisted that, if the psychiatrists continued to request that this arrangement should apply, they should prepare a document setting out in detail their reasons and the benefits that they believed would result from it. To this he would add a document stating, on behalf of himself and the clinical nurses, their reasons (of principle and practicability) why this method was considered inappropriate.

Faced with this insistence that reasons for the requirement be stated in writing, the psychiatrists withdrew the instruction.

Study B19: Discussion

Clause 10 of the Code of Professional Conduct and the supplementary advisory document (see Appendix 2) are relevant to this case. Although emphasising the importance of confidentiality, the latter document states that it is a rule with certain exceptions. Those exceptions focus around a 'public interest' justification.

In this case, after weighing up the risks and benefits on each side, the nurse decided to inform the police.

Study B20: Discussion

This practice nurse had to decide whether this set of circumstances might possibly be regarded as one of the rare exceptions in which a breach of the important principle of confidentiality could be justified. She realised that such justification must depend on a public interest argument. She decided, on balance, to do nothing but to enjoy spending the money received from the insurance company.

Appendix 2

Guidelines for Professional Practice

Preamble

The UKCC has produced this booklet to provide a guide for reflection on the statements within the Code of Professional Conduct. For students and those of you who are new to the professions, we hope that you find it useful; others of you may be very familiar with the guidance provided. This booklet has been produced to help to reflect on the many challenges that face us in day-to-day practice. The booklet should be read as a whole and care should be taken to use each section in the context of all the guidance provided. It is important that time is taken to read and consider the whole document. You may find yourself in a crisis when there is no opportunity to reach for a book. At these times, you may need guidance offered to make the professional judgement needed for that specific situation.

Once you have read the booklet, you will be able to dip into the relevant sections and we hope that you will use it regularly and reflect on the many subjects covered. Throughout this booklet, many general ethical and legal issues have been covered. However, it is important that you get to know the specific circumstances, safeguards, policies and procedures needed to provide treatment or care relevant to your area of practice.

The development of these guidelines has been a consultative process with input from individuals with different employment, education, consumer and practice backgrounds. It has been produced in order to replace and update the information provided in the following three documents; *Exercising Accountability* (March 1989), *Confidentiality* (April 1987) and *Advertising by Registered Nurses, Midwives and Health Visitors* (March 1985).

With the many challenges facing nurses, midwives and health visitors and the speed in which practice changes, we acknowledge that these guidelines for professional practice will require regular review. We will formally review the contents by June 1998 and, in the meantime, would welcome any comments you have. These should be sent to the Professional Officer, Ethics, at the UKCC's address.

Introduction

(1) The UKCC's responsibilities are set out in the Nurses, Midwives and Health Visitors Acts for 1979 and 1992 and our main responsibility is to protect the

interests of the public. To do this, we set standards for education, training and professional conduct for registered nurses, midwives and health visitors (registered practitioners). The motto on our coat of arms – 'care, protect, honour' – reflects these responsibilities. We hope that this booklet will help you to:

- 'care' in a way that reflects your code of professional conduct (the UKCC Code of Professional Conduct 1992);
- 'protect' patients and clients and
- 'honour' your responsibilities as a registered practitioner.

(2) With so many codes and charters about, it is easy to be confused about how they relate to your professional and personal life. The Code of Professional Conduct was drawn up by the UKCC under the powers of the Nurses, Midwives and Health Visitors Act 1979 to give advice to registered practitioners. This code sets out:

- the value of registered practitioners;
- your responsibilities to represent and protect the interests of patients and clients; and
- what is expected of you.

(3) The role of the UKCC in protecting the public is firstly to maintain a register of people who are recommended to be suitable practitioners and who have demonstrated knowledge and skill through a qualification registered with the UKCC. Secondly, we can remove people from that register either because they are seriously ill or because a charge of misconduct has been proven against them. The code is used as the standard against which complaints are considered.

(4) This booklet gives guidance on all sixteen clauses of the code. It deals with areas such as consent, truthfulness, advocacy and autonomy. It cannot deal with every conflict which a registered practitioner may face. We recognise that professional practice and decision-making are not straightforward. The circumstances we work under are always changing. The way we work must be sensitive and relevant and must meet the needs of patients and clients. We must be able to adjust our practice to changing circumstances, taking into consideration local procedures, policies and cultural differences.

Accountability – answering for your actions

(5) As a registered practitioner, you hold a position of responsibility and other people rely on you. You are professionally accountable to the UKCC, as well as having a contractual accountability to your employer and accountability to the law for your actions. The Code of Professional Conduct sets out your professional accountability – to whom you must answer and how. The code begins with the statement that:

> 'Each registered nurse, midwife and health visitor shall act, at all times, in such a manner as to: safeguard and promote the interests of individual

patients and clients; serve the interests of society; justify public trust and confidence and uphold and enhance the good standing and reputation of the professions.'

Each clause of the code begins with the statement that:

'As a registered nurse, midwife or health visitor, you are personally accountable for your practice and, in the exercise of your professional accountability, must...'

No one else can answer for you and it is no defence to say that you were acting on someone else's orders.

(6) In exercising your professional accountability, there may be conflict between the interests of a patient or client, the health or social care team and society. This is especially so if health care resources are limited. Whatever decisions you take and judgements you make, you must be able to justify your actions.

(7) Accountability is an integral part of professional practice, as in the course of practice you have to make judgements in a wide variety of circumstances. Professional accountability is fundamentally concerned with weighing up the interests of patients and clients in complex situations, using professional knowledge, judgement and skills to make a decision and enabling you to account for the decision made. Neither the Code of Professional Conduct nor this booklet seek to state the circumstances in which accountability has to be exercised, but instead they provide principles to aid your decision making.

(8) If you delegate work to someone who is not registered with the UKCC, your accountability is to make sure that the person who does the work is able to do it and that appropriate levels of supervision or support are in place.

(9) The first four clauses of the code make sure that you put the interests of patients, clients and the public before your own interests and those of your professional colleagues. They are as follows:

'As a registered nurse, midwife or health visitor, you are personally accountable for your practice and, in the exercise of your professional accountability, must...

1 act always in such a manner as to promote and safeguard the interests and well-being of patients and clients;
2 ensure that no action or omission on your part, or within your sphere of responsibility, is detrimental to the interests, condition or safety of patients and clients;
3 maintain and improve your professional knowledge and competence;
4 acknowledge any limitations in your knowledge and competence and decline any duties or responsibilities unless able to perform them in a safe and skilled manner;'

(10) The code does not cover the specific circumstances in which you make decisions and judgements. It presents important themes and principles which you must apply to all areas of your work.

Duty of care

(11) You have both a legal and a professional duty to care for patients and clients. In law, the courts could find a registered practitioner negligent if a person suffers harm because he or she failed to care for them properly. Professionally, the UKCC's Professional Conduct Committee could find a registered practitioner guilty of misconduct and remove them from the register if he or she failed to care properly for a patient or client, even though they suffered no harm.

(12) Lord Atkin defined the duty of care when he gave judgement in the case of *Donoghue v. Stephenson* (House of Lords) (1932). He said that:

> 'You must take reasonable care to avoid acts or omissions which you can reasonably foresee would be likely to injure your neighbour. Who, then, in the law is my neighbour? The answer seems to be persons who are so closely and directly affected by my act that I ought to have them in contemplation as being so affected when I am directing my mind to the acts or omissions which are called in question.'

How circumstances can affect your duty of care

(13) If there is a complaint against you, the UKCC's Professional Conduct Committee and possibly the courts would decide whether you took proper care. When they do this, they must consider whether what you did was reasonable in all the circumstances.

(14) The following examples show how the duty of care changes according to the circumstances. Each example shows a skilled adult intensive care nurse in a different situation.

Example 1

The nurse is on duty in the intensive care unit when a patient suffers a cardiac arrest.

Here, it is reasonable to expect the nurse to care for the patient as competently as any experienced intensive care unit nurse.

Example 2

The nurse is walking along a hospital corridor and finds a woman completely alone giving birth.

In this situation, it is not reasonable to expect the nurse to care for the woman as a midwife would. But it is reasonable to expect the nurse to call a midwife or obstetrician and to stay with the woman until appropriate help arrives.

Example 3

The nurse is walking along a street and comes across a person injured in a road traffic accident.

In this situation, the nurse does not have a legal duty to stop and care for the injured person. But if she does, she then takes on a legal duty to care for the person properly. In these circumstances, it is reasonable to expect her to care for the person to the best of her skill and knowledge. Although the nurse has no legal duty to stop and give care in this example, she does have a professional duty. The Code of Professional Conduct places a professional duty upon her at all times. However, in this situation it could be reasonable to expect the nurse to do no more than comfort and support the injured person.

What is reasonable?

(15) The courts and the Professional Conduct Committee must decide whether your actions were reasonable. The case of *Bolam v. Friern Hospital Management Committee* (1957) produced this test of what is reasonable:

> 'The test is the standard of the ordinary skilled man exercising and professing to have that special skill. A man need not possess the highest expert skill at the risk of being found negligent ... it is sufficient if he exercises the skill of an ordinary competent man exercising that particular art.'

(16) This test is usually called the Bolam test. Although the case concerned a doctor, the Bolam test can be used to examine the actions of any professional person. The case of *Wilsher v. Essex AHA* (1988) set the standard of reasonable care to be expected of students and junior staff. The standard is that of a reasonably competent practitioner and not that of a student or junior. You have a duty to ensure that the care which you delegate is carried out at a reasonably competent standard. This means that you remain accountable for the delegation of the work and for ensuring that the person who does the work is able to do it. The Code of Professional Conduct provides principles which you can apply to any situation. If you use these principles, you will be able to carry out your legal and professional duty of care.

Withdrawing care to protect the public and yourself

(17) There may be circumstances of conflict where the registered practitioner may consider withdrawing his or her care. A situation like this might occur if the registered practitioner fears physical violence or if there are health and safety hazards involved in providing care. There may be other situations where the registered practitioner may seek support or consider withdrawing care, for example due to sexual or racial harassment. Any decision to withdraw care has to be taken very carefully and you should first discuss, if possible, the matter with managers, the patient's or client's family and, if appropriate and wherever possible, the patient or client themselves. In certain circumstances, you may need help to make sure that the public are safe. If possible, you should discuss this with other members of the health care team. However, in areas of practice where violence may occur more frequently, such as in some areas of mental health care and in accident and emergency departments, there must be protocols to deal with these situations. Appropriate training and on-call support arrangements should also be available. In all cases, you should make a record of the fact that you withdrew care so that if your actions or decisions are questioned, you can justify them.

Patient and client advocacy and autonomy

(18) Recognising a patient's or client's right to choose is clearly outlined in clauses 1 and 5 of the code. Although the words advocacy and autonomy are not specifically used, it is this section which states the registered practitioner's role in these respects. The code states that:

> 'As a registered nurse, midwife or health visitor, you are personally accountable for your practice and, in the exercise of your professional accountability, must...
>
> 1 ... act always in such a manner as to promote and safeguard the interests and well-being of patients and clients; (advocacy)...
>
> 5 ... work in an open and co-operative manner with patients, clients and their families, foster their independence and recognise and respect their involvement in the planning and delivery of care;' (autonomy)

(19) The registered practitioner must not practise in a way which assumes that only they know what is best for the patient or client, as this can only create a dependence and interfere with the patient's or client's right to choose. Advocacy is concerned with promoting and protecting the interests of patients or clients, many of whom may be vulnerable and incapable of protecting their own interests and who may be without the support of family or friends. You can do this by providing information and making the patient or client feel confident that he or she can make their own decisions. Advocacy also involves providing support if the patient refuses treatment/care or withdraws their consent. Other health care professionals, families, legal advisers, voluntary agencies and advocates appointed by the courts may also be involved in safeguarding the interests of patients and clients.

(20) Respect for patients' and clients' autonomy means that you should respect the choices they make concerning their own lives. Clause 5 of the code outlines your professional role in promoting patient/client independence. This means discussing with them any proposed treatment or care so that they can decide whether to refuse or accept that treatment or care. This information should enable the patient or client to decide what is in their own best interests.

(21) Registered practitioners must respect patients' and clients' rights to take part in decisions about their care. You must use your professional judgement, often in conjunction with colleagues, to decide when a patient or client is capable of making an informed decision about his or her treatment and care. If possible, the patient or client should be able to make a choice about his or her care, even if this means that they may refuse care. You must make sure that all decisions are based on relevant knowledge. The patient's or client's right to agree to or to refuse treatment and care may change in law depending on their age and health (refer to the section on consent on pages 189–91). Particular attention to the legal position of children must be given, as their right to give consent or refuse treatment or care varies in different parts of the United Kingdom and depending on their age.

Communicating

(22) Communication is an essential part of good practice. The patient or client can only make an informed choice if he or she is given clear information at every stage of care. You also need to listen to the patient or client. Listening is a vital part of communication. Effective communication relies on all our skills. Building a trusting relationship will greatly improve care and help to reduce anxiety and stress for patients and clients, their families and their carers. For effective communication, you may need to consult other colleagues with specialist knowledge, or you may need the services of interpreters to make sure that information is understood. It is important to create an environment for good communication so that you can build a relationship of trust with the patient or client. Employers should recognise the importance of communication when they plan staffing structures and levels.

(23) To ensure that you gain the trust of your patients and clients, you should recognise them as equal partners, use language that is familiar to them and make sure that they understand the information you are giving. Your records must also be clear, legible and accessible to the patient or client, as outlined in the UKCC's document *Standards for Records and Record Keeping* and under the terms of the Data Protection Act 1984 and the Access to Health Records Act 1990. Written communication is as important as verbal communication.

Truthfulness

(24) Patients and clients have a legal right to information about their condition; registered practitioners providing care have a professional duty to provide such information. A patient or client who wants information is entitled to an honest answer. There may be rare occasions when a person's condition and the likely effect of information given at a specific time might lead you to be selective (although never untruthful) about the information you give. Any decision you make about what information to give must be in the best interests of the patient or client.

(25) There is potential for disagreement or even conflict between different professionals and relatives over giving information to a patient or client. When discussing these matters with colleagues or relatives, you must stress that your personal accountability is firstly to the patient and client. Any patient or client can feel relatively powerless when they do not have full knowledge about their care or treatment. Giving patients and clients information helps to empower them. For this reason, the importance of telling the truth cannot be overestimated. If patients or clients do not want to know the truth, it should not be forced upon them. You must be sensitive to their needs and must make sure that your communication is effective. The patient or client must be given a choice in the matter. To deny them that choice is to deny their rights and so diminish their dignity and independence.

Consent

(26) You must obtain consent before you can give any treatment or care. The patient's or client's decision whether or not to agree to treatment must be based on adequate information so that they can make up their mind. It is important that this information is shared freely with the patient or client, in an accessible way and in appropriate circumstances. In emergency situations, where treatment is necessary to preserve life and the patient or client cannot make a decision (for example because they are unconscious), the law allows you to provide treatment without the patient's or client's consent, always acting in the best interests of the patient or client. You should also know that if the patient or client is an adult, consent from relatives is not sufficient on its own to protect you in the event of challenge, as nobody has the right to give consent on behalf of another adult.

(27) When the patient or client is told about proposed treatment and care, it is important that you give the information in a sensitive and understandable way and that you give the patient or client enough time to consider it and ask questions if they wish. It is not safe to assume that the patient or client has enough knowledge, even about basic treatment, for them to make an informed choice without an explanation. You must respect the patient's or client's decision, regardless of whether he or she agrees to or refuses treatment.

(28) It is essential that you give the patient or client adequate information so that he or she can make a meaningful decision. If a patient or client feels that the information they received was insufficient, they could make a complaint to the UKCC or take legal action. Most legal action is in the form of an allegation of negligence. In exceptional cases, for example where a patient's or client's consent was obtained by deception or where not enough information was given, this could result in an allegation of battery (or civil assault in Scotland). However, only in the most extreme cases is criminal law likely to be involved.

Who should obtain consent?

(29) It is important that the person proposing to perform a procedure should obtain consent, although there may be some urgent situations where another practitioner can do so. Sometimes you may not be responsible for obtaining a patient's or client's consent as, although you are caring for the patient or client, you would not actually be carrying out the procedure. However, you are often best placed to know about the emotions, concerns and views of the patient or client and may be best able to judge what information is needed so that it is understood. With this in mind, you should tell other members of the health care team if you are concerned about the patient's or client's understanding of the procedure or treatment, for example, due to language difficulties.

Types of consent

(30) Although the most important aspect of obtaining consent is providing and sharing information, the patient or client may demonstrate their decision in a

number of ways. If they agree to treatment and care, they may do so verbally, in writing or by implying (by co-operating) that they agree. Equally a patient or client may withdraw or refuse consent in the same way. Verbal consent, or consent by implication, will be enough evidence in most cases. You should obtain written consent if the treatment or care is risky, lengthy or complex. This written consent stands as a record that discussions have taken place and of the patient's or client's choice. If a patient or client refuses treatment, making a written record of this is just as important. You should make sure that a summary of the discussions and decisions is placed in the patient's or client's records.

When consent is refused

(31) Legally, a competent adult patient can either give or refuse consent to treatment, even if that refusal will shorten their life. Therefore you must respect the patient's refusal just as much as you would their consent. You must make sure that the patient is fully informed and, when necessary, involve other members of the health care team. As before, you should make sure that a summary of the discussions and decisions is placed in the patient's or client's records.

(32) Increasingly, the law and professional bodies are also recognising the power of advanced directives or living wills. These are documents made in advance of a particular condition arising and they show the patient's or client's treatment choices, including the decision not to accept further treatment in certain circumstances. Although not necessarily legally binding, they can provide very useful information about the wishes of a patient or client who is now unable to make a decision and therefore should be respected.

Consent of people under 16

(33) If the patient or client is under the age of 16 (a minor), you must be aware of local protocols and legislation that affect their care or treatment. Consent of patients or clients under 16 is very complex, so you may need to seek local, legal or membership organisation advice. Some of the laws relating to a minor's consent have been referenced at the back of this booklet.

Consent of people who are mentally incapacitated

(34) It is important that the principles governing consent are applied just as vigorously to all forms of care with people who are mentally incapacitated as with a competent adult. A patient or client may be described as mentally incapacitated for a number of reasons. There may be temporary reasons such as sedatory medicines or longer term reasons such as mental illness, coma or unconsciousness.

(35) When a patient or client is considered incapable of providing consent, or where the wishes of a mentally incapacitated patient or client appear to be contrary to the interests of that person, you should be involved in assessing their care or treatment. You should consult relevant people close to the patient or client, but respect any previous instructions the patient or client gave.

(36) In some cases of legal incapacity, such as when a patient is in a persistent vegetative state, certain decisions will need court authority. Court authority may also be necessary or desirable in decisions concerning selective non-treatment of handicapped infants, dealing with certain circumstances of neonate care or sterilisation of a mentally handicapped individual.

Mental Health Acts

(37) If you are involved in the care or treatment of patients or clients detained under statutory powers in the Mental Health Acts, you must get to know the circumstances and safeguards needed for providing treatment and care without consent.

Making concerns known

(38) Employers have a duty to provide the resources needed for patient and client care, but the numerous requests to the UKCC for advice on this subject indicate that the environment in which care is provided is not always adequate. You may find yourself unable to provide good care because of a lack of adequate resources. Also, you may be afraid to speak out for fear of losing your job. However, if you do not report your concerns, you may be in breach of the Code of Professional Conduct. You may also have concerns over inappropriate behaviour by a colleague and feel it necessary to make your concerns known. You will need to report your concerns to the appropriate person or authority, depending on the type of concerns. You may feel it necessary to discuss these decisions with other colleagues or a membership organisation.

(39) The clauses of the code which relate specifically to these issues are numbers 11, 12 and 13:

> 'As a registered nurse, midwife and health visitor, you are personally accountable for your practice and, in the exercise of your professional accountability, must...
>
> 11 report to an appropriate person or authority, having regard to the physical, psychological and social effects on patients and clients, any circumstances in the environment of care which could jeopardise standards of practice;
>
> 12 report to an appropriate person or authority any circumstances in which safe and appropriate care for patients and clients cannot be provided;
>
> 13 report to an appropriate person or authority where it appears that the health or safety of colleagues is at risk, as such circumstances may compromise standards of practice and care;'

(40) These clauses give advice on the minimum action to be taken. This will help to make sure that those who manage resources and staff have all the information they need to provide an adequate and appropriate standard of care. You must not be deterred from reporting your concerns, even if you believe that resources are not available or that no action will be taken. You should make your report

verbally and/or in writing and, where available, follow local procedures. The manager (who may also be registered with us) should assess the report and communicate it to senior managers where appropriate. This is important because if, subsequently, any complaint is made about the registered practitioners involved in providing care, this may require senior managers to justify their actions if inadequate resources are seen to affect the situation.

(41) As outlined in clauses 11, 12 and 13 of the code, the registered practitioner's role is to make sure that safe and appropriate care is provided. This means:

- promoting staff support throughout health care settings;
- telling senior colleagues about unacceptable standards;
- supporting and advising colleagues at risk;
- reporting circumstances in the environment which could jeopardise standards of practice;
- making sure that local procedures are in place, challenged and/or changed;
- being aware of new codes, charters and registration body guidelines;
- keeping accurate records and
- when necessary, obtaining guidance on how to present information to management.

Working together

(42) The UKCC recognises the complexity of health care and stresses the need to appreciate the contribution of professional health care staff, students, supporting staff and also voluntary and independent agencies. Providing care is a multi-professional, multi-agency activity which, in order to be effective, must be based on mutual understanding, trust, respect and co-operation. Patients and clients are equal partners in their care and therefore have the right to be involved in the health care team's decisions.

(43) Under clause 6 and clause 14 of the Code of Professional Conduct:

> 'As a registered nurse, midwife or health visitor, you are personally accountable for your practice and, in the exercise of your professional accountability, must...
>
> 6 work in a collaborative and co-operative manner with health care professionals and others involved in providing care, and recognise and respect their particular contributions within the care team;...
>
> 14 assist professional colleagues, in the context of your own knowledge, experience and sphere of responsibility, to develop their professional competence and assist others in the care team, including informal carers, to contribute safely to a degree appropriate to their roles;'

These clauses emphasise the importance of support and co-operation and also the importance of avoiding disputes and promoting good relationships and a spirit of co-operation and mutual respect within the health and social care team. It is clearly impossible for any one profession to possess all the knowledge, skills and resources needed to meet the total health care needs of society. Good care should be the product of a good team.

(44) Good team work is important but co-operation and collaboration are not always easily achieved, for example, if:

- individual members of the team have their own specific and separate objectives or
- one member of the team tries to adopt a dominant role without considering the opinions, knowledge and skills of its other members.

In such circumstances, achieving good team work needs hard work and negotiation between all the health care professionals involved. In all the discussions, it is important to stress that the interests of the patient or client must come first.

(45) Discrimination has no place in health care. This means making sure that equal opportunities policies are in place, challenged and/or changed and ensuring that no one has to endure racial or sexual harassment. Each member of a team is entitled to equality and must not be discriminated against because of gender, age, race, disability, sexuality, culture or religious beliefs. There needs to be effective communication and team work to make sure these principles are not neglected.

Conscientious objection

(46) In today's developing health service, you may find yourself in situations which you find very uncomfortable. There may be many circumstances in which a practitioner, due to personal morality or religious beliefs, will not wish to be involved in a certain type of treatment or care. Clause 8 of the Code of Professional Conduct states that:

> 'As a registered nurse, midwife or health visitor, you are personally accountable for your practice and, in the exercise of your professional accountability, must...
>
> 8 report to an appropriate person or authority, at the earliest possible time, any conscientious objection which may be relevant to your professional practice;'

(47) In law, you have the right conscientiously to object to take part in care in only two areas. These are the Abortion Act 1967 (Scotland, England and Wales), which gives you the right to refuse to take part in an abortion, and the Human Fertilisation and Embryology Act 1990, which gives you the right to refuse to participate in technological procedures to achieve conception and pregnancy.

(48) However, in an emergency, you would be expected to provide care. You should carefully consider whether or not to accept employment in an area which carries out treatment or procedures to which you object. If, however, a situation arises in which you do not want to take part in a form of treatment or care, then it is important that you declare your objection in time for managers to make alternative arrangements. In certain circumstances, this may mean providing

counselling for the staff involved in these decisions. You do not have the right to refuse to take part in emergency treatment.

(49) Refusing to be involved in the care of patients because of their condition or behaviour is unacceptable. The UKCC expects all registered practitioners to be non-judgmental when providing care. This is one of the issues addressed by clause 7 of the code, which states that:

> 'As a registered nurse, midwife or health visitor, you are personally accountable for your practice and, in the exercise of your professional accountability, must...
>
> 7 recognise and respect the uniqueness and dignity of each patient and client, and respect their need for care, irrespective of their ethnic origin, religious beliefs, personal attributes, the nature of their health problems or any other factor;'

Confidentiality

(50) To trust another person with private and personal information about yourself is a significant matter. If the person to whom that information is given is a nurse, midwife or health visitor, the patient or client has a right to believe that this information, given in confidence, will only be used for the purposes for which it was given and will not be released to others without their permission. The death of a patient or client does not give you the right to break confidentiality.

(51) Clause 10 of the Code of Professional Conduct addresses this subject directly. It states that:

> 'As a registered nurse, midwife or health visitor, you are personally accountable for your practice and, in the exercise of your professional accountability, must...
>
> 10 protect all confidential information concerning patients and clients obtained in the course of professional practice and make disclosures only with consent, where required by the order of a court or where you can justify disclosure in the wider public interest;'

Confidentiality should only be broken in exceptional circumstances and should only occur after careful consideration that you can justify your action.

(52) It is impractical to obtain the consent of the patient or client every time you need to share information with other health professionals or other staff involved in the health care of that patient or client. What is important is that the patient or client understands that some information may be made available to others involved in the delivery of their care. However, the patient or client must know who the information will be shared with.

(53) Patients and clients have a right to know the standards of confidentiality maintained by those providing their care and these standards should be made known by the health professional at the first point of contact. These standards of confidentiality can be reinforced by leaflets and posters where the health care is being delivered.

Providing information

(54) You always need to obtain the explicit consent of a patient or client before you disclose specific information and you must make sure that the patient or client can make an informed response as to whether that information can be disclosed.

(55) Disclosure of information occurs:

- with the consent of the patient or client;
- without the consent of the patient or client when the disclosure is required by law or by order of a court and
- without the consent of the patient or client when the disclosure is considered to be necessary in the public interest.

(56) The public interest means the interests of an individual, or groups of individuals or of society as a whole, and would, for example, cover matters such as serious crime, child abuse, drug trafficking or other activities which place others at serious risk.

(57) There is no statutory right to confidentiality but an aggrieved individual can sue through a civil court alleging that confidentiality was broken.

(58) The situation that causes most problems is when your decision to withhold confidential information or give it to a third party has serious consequences. The information may have been given to you in the strictest confidence by a patient or client or by a colleague. You could also discover the information in the course of your work.

(59) You may sometimes be under pressure to release information but you must realise that you will be held accountable for this. In all cases where you deliberately release information in what you believe to be the best interests of the public, your decision must be justified. In some circumstances, such as accident and emergency admissions where the police are involved, it may be appropriate to involve senior staff if you do not feel that you are able to deal with the situation alone.

(60) The above circumstances can be particularly stressful, especially if vulnerable groups are concerned, as releasing information may mean that a third party becomes involved, as in the case of children or those with learning difficulties.

(61) You should always discuss the matter fully with other professional colleagues and, if appropriate, consult the UKCC or a membership organisation before making a decision to release information without a patient's permission. There will often be significant consequences which you must consider carefully before you make the decision to withhold or release information. Having made a decision, you should write down the reasons either in the appropriate record or in a special note that can be kept in a separate file (outlined in the UKCC's booklet *Standards for Records and Record Keeping*). You then have written justification for the action which you took if this becomes necessary and you can also review the decision later in the light of future developments.

Ownership of and access to records

(62) Organisations which employ professional staff who make records are the legal owners of these records, but that does not give anyone in that organisation the

legal right of access to the information in those records. However, the patient or client can ask to see their records, whether they are written down or on computer. This is as a result of the Data Protection Act 1984, Access Modification (Health) Order 1987 and the Access to Health Records Act 1990.

(63) The contracts of employment of all employees not directly involved with patients but who have access to or handle confidential records should contain clauses which emphasise the principles of confidentiality and state the disciplinary action which could result if these principles are not met.

(64) As far as computer-held records are concerned, you must be satisfied that as far as possible, the methods you use for recording information are secure. You must also find out which categories of staff have access to records to which they are expected to contribute important personal and confidential information. Local procedures must include ways of checking whether a record is authentic when there is no written signature. All records must clearly indicate the identity of the person who made that record. As more patient and client records are moved and linked between health care settings by computer, you will have to be vigilant in order to make sure that patient or client confidentiality is not broken. This means trying to ensure that the systems used are protected from inappropriate access within your direct area of practice, for example ensuring that personal access codes are kept secure.

(65) The Computer Misuse Act 1990 came into force to secure computer programs and data against unauthorised access or alteration. Authorised users have permission to use certain programs and data. If those users go beyond what is permitted, this is a criminal offence. The Act makes provision for accidentally exceeding your permission and covers fraud, extortion and blackmail.

(66) Where access to information contained on a computer filing system is available to members of staff who are not registered practitioners, or health professionals governed by similar ethical principles, an important clause concerning confidentiality should appear within their contracts of employment (outlined in the UKCC's position statement *Confidentiality: use of computers*, 1994).

(67) Those who receive confidential information from a patient or client should advise them that the information will be given to the registered practitioner involved in their care. If necessary, this may also include other professionals in the health and social work fields. Registered practitioners must make sure that, where possible, the storage and movement of records within the health care setting does not put the confidentiality of patient information at risk.

Access to records for teaching, research and audit

(68) If patients' or clients' records need to be used to help students gain the knowledge and skills which they require, the same principles of confidentiality apply to the information. This also applies to those engaged in research and audit. The manager of the health care setting is responsible for the security of the information contained in these records and for making sure that access to the information is closely supervised. The person providing the training will be responsible for making sure that students understand the need for confidentiality and the need to follow local procedures for handling and storing

records. The patient or client should know about the individual having access to their records and should be able to refuse that access if they wish.

(69) In summary, the following principles concerning confidentiality apply:

- a patient or client has the right to expect that information given in confidence will be used only for the purpose for which it was given and will not be released to others without their permission;
- you should recognise each patient's or client's right to have information about themselves kept secure and private;
- if it is appropriate to share information gained in the course of your work with other health or social work practitioners, you must make sure that as far as is reasonable, the information will be kept in strict professional confidence and be used only for the purpose for which the information was given;
- you are responsible for any decision which you make to release confidential information because you think that this is in the public's best interest;
- if you choose to break confidentiality because you believe that this is in the public's best interest, you must have considered the situation carefully enough to justify that decision and
- you should not deliberately break confidentiality other than in exceptional circumstances.

Advertising and sponsorship

(70) Clause 16 of the UKCC's Code of Professional Conduct addresses the subject of the promotion of commercial goods or services. It states that:

> 'As a registered nurse, midwife or health visitor, you are personally accountable for your practice and, in the exercise of your professional accountability, must . . .
>
> 16 ensure that your registration status is not used in the promotion of commercial products or services, declare any financial or other interests in relevant organisations providing such goods or services and ensure that your professional judgement is not influenced by any commercial considerations.'

(71) Patients or clients and their relatives or friends are often anxious when attending hospitals and other health care facilities. The environment of care should help to promote good health, healing and recovery and not be one of commercial advertising.

(72) Clause 16 does not intend to prevent registered practitioners employed in positions such as the matron of a private nursing home or as a representative of a pharmaceutical company, or who are offering their professional services privately, from using their registration status on items such as business cards and headed note paper.

(73) However, if a practitioner has a direct financial or other direct interest in an organisation providing commercial goods or services, for example, a ward sister who is discharging a patient to a nursing home owned and run by herself or one of her relatives, then that practitioner must make her interests known.

(74) It is also unacceptable for registered practitioners to carry commercial advertising or promotional material on their uniforms.

(75) Under the Code of Professional Conduct, registered practitioners must protect the interests of patients and clients, be worthy of public trust and confidence and avoid using professional qualifications in ways which might compromise the independence of professional judgements upon which patients and clients rely. The vulnerability of patients and clients is reflected by these elements of the code, which also indicate the importance of trust between a registered practitioner and a patient as well as the expectation that the registered practitioner will respond to the patient's needs unconditionally.

Sponsorship

(76) Funding for some posts, projects or services is sometimes offered by companies, some of which have a commercial interest in matters associated with health care. Sponsorship arrangements which affect the professional judgement of registered practitioners and patient or client choice should be brought to the attention of those who provide health care services.

(77) Students on pre-registration and post-registration courses often need sponsorship to carry out their study, especially for overseas study visits. The decision to accept sponsorship must be made by the individual, taking account of the appropriateness of the support offered.

Receiving gifts

(78) You may be offered gifts, favours or hospitality from patients or clients during the course of or after a period of care or treatment. The Code of Professional Conduct states that:

> 'As a registered nurse, midwife and health visitor, you are personally accountable for your practice and, in the exercise of your professional accountability must...
>
> 15 refuse any gift, favour or hospitality from patients or clients currently in your care which might be interpreted as seeking to exert influence to obtain preferential consideration;'

The important principle is not that the registered practitioner never receives gifts or favours but that they could never be interpreted as being given by the patient or client in return for preferential treatment.

Complementary and alternative therapies

(79) Complementary therapies are gaining popularity and finding a more substantial place in health care. It is vitally important that you ensure that the introduction of any of these therapies to your practice is always in the best interests and safety of the patients and clients. Clause 9 of the code outlines your privileged relationship with patients and clients:

> 'As a registered nurse, midwife and health visitor, you are personally accountable for your practice and, in the exercise of your professional accountability must . . .
>
> 9 avoid any abuse of your privileged relationship with patients and clients and of the privileged access allowed to their person, property, residence or workplace;'

The registered practitioner therefore must be convinced of the relevance and accountability of the therapy being used and must be able to justify using it in a particular circumstance, especially when using the therapy as part of professional practice. It should also be part of professional team work to discuss the use of complementary therapies with medical and other members of the health care team caring for the particular patient or client.

(80) Some registered practitioners, who successfully complete courses in complementary or alternative therapies not usually associated with their professional practice, quote their registration status when advertising their services. The UKCC believes that a person's registration status should not be needed to support a complementary or alternative therapy course or qualification if the course is valid and credible. However, if it is a registered practitioner's registered status that gives credibility to the qualification, then the registered practitioner must use their own judgement and discretion to make sure that they are not misleading the public.

(81) If a complaint is made against you, we can call you to account for any activities carried out outside conventional practice. You should carefully consider the content and status of any courses which you undertake and how you promote yourself.

Research and audit

(82) Increasing numbers of registered practitioners are carrying out, or are involved in, research or audit. The results might improve practice, help to audit an aspect of clinical services, inform policy or be part of a graduate or postgraduate qualification. Other practitioners are employed or involved with clinical trials which focus on new treatments, new technology or improvements to patient care.

(83) If you are involved in these activities, issues often arise which you need to consider. Is the research ethical? Is your role appropriate? Has the Local Research Ethics Committee (LREC) given its approval? Has local management given their approval? What is the make-up of the LREC? Are there registered practitioners on the LREC?

Types of research

(84) The range of research carried out varies greatly. Outlined below are some of the types of research that are used in the health care setting.

Projects

(85) An increasing number of students are being asked to do project work for diplomas or undergraduate degrees. Many educational institutions recommend that their diploma or undergraduate students do not become involved in clinically-based research.

(86) As the number of these projects increases, contact with patients or clients might be refused. This is quite reasonable, as the care and comfort of patients or clients must always be considered. Projects by registered practitioners may be prompted by developments at clinical level, by involvement in practice development units or as a result of participating in clinical supervision.

Higher degrees

(87) Research for postgraduate degrees is supervised and guided throughout. It is important to gain approval for research in clinical areas from management in addition to consulting the local LREC before starting the work.

Other research work and clinical research trials

(88) Research activities intended to benefit patient care or investigate practice are carried out by a wide range of clinicians, academics and others. Registered practitioners may be involved in this work as part of their job, because of academic interest or in response to a perceived or expressed need.

(89) Contracts of employment specify how practitioners must work. They do not always cover concerns about the ethics of research, confidentiality, consent or other issues. Under European Community Directive 91/507/EEC, all elements of clinical trials carried out within the European Union must adhere to the guidelines on good clinical practice for trials on medical protocols in the EU. These guidelines provide a useful framework for nurses, midwives and health visitors to use when they are involved in research work.

(90) If there is contact with patients or clients, it is important for you to discuss the benefits of the work with the appropriate manager. You must be certain that approval from the LREC is obtained. Repeated requests for patients and clients to fill in questionnaires or to be interviewed can be intrusive and potentially disruptive to care. For this reason, the views of patients, clients, and their associates will assist in determining prospective compliance.

Criteria for safe and ethical conduct of research

(91) You must always refer to the UKCC's Code of Professional Conduct and The Scope of Professional Practice. These documents provide the framework for all actions of registered nurses, midwives and health visitors.

(92) As well as using these documents, you need to be sure that the research or clinical trial you are carrying out meets specific criteria. These are that:

- the project must be approved by the LREC;
- management approval must be gained where necessary;

- arrangements for obtaining consent must be clearly understood by all those involved;
- confidentiality must be maintained;
- patients must not be exposed to unacceptable risks;
- patients should be included in the development of proposed projects where appropriate;
- accurate records must be kept and
- research questions need to be well structured and aimed at producing clearly anticipated care or service outcomes and benefits.

(93) You need to consider these criteria before submitting a research proposal to a LREC. You are expected to participate fully in the design process and this includes raising legitimate concerns when they arise. If no LREC exists in your area, it is important to refer to local policy for research.

Audit

(94) Audit seeks to improve practice and treatment and to reduce risk by the systematic review of the process and outcome of care and treatment and by the evaluation of records and other data. There are occasions when contact with patients and clients, carers or relatives is necessary and therefore LREC clearance may be required. Consideration of the other points highlighted above is recommended.

Conclusion

(95) We have produced this booklet to help you in your professional practice. It would be impossible to discuss all the issues faced by registered practitioners. Answers are not always straightforward. The Code of Professional Conduct and The Scope of Professional Practice apply to all registered practitioners and the interests of the public, patients and clients are of the greatest importance. You should also remember that being accountable and working with those who provide care is the foundation upon which the best standards are achieved. With the many challenges facing nurses, midwives and health visitors and the speed in which practice changes, it is acknowledged that these guidelines for professional practice will require regular review. We will formally review these guidelines by June 1998 and, in the meantime, would welcome any comments which you may have. Comments on this booklet should be sent to the Professional Officer, Ethics, at the UKCC's address.

(96) In producing this booklet, we have been greatly helped by comments from representatives of practice, education, medical, professional, membership and consumer organisations. We have tried to produce the booklet in a form that is easily accessible in order to aid professional judgement and to outline basic principles.

(97) If you need further information or advice, please contact our team of professional officers at the:

Standards Promotion Directorate
United Kingdom Central Council
for Nursing, Midwifery and Health Visiting
23 Portland Place
London W1N 4JT

Telephone: 0171 637 7181
Fax: 0171 436 2924

Documents relevant to these guidelines

(1) *Code of Professional Conduct*, UKCC, 1992
(2) *The Scope of Professional Practice*, UKCC, 1992
(3) *Midwives Rules*, UKCC, 1993
(4) *The Midwife's Code of Practice*, UKCC, 1994
(5) *Standards for Records and Record Keeping*, UKCC, 1993
(6) *Standards for the Administration of Medicines*, UKCC, 1992
(7) *Confidentiality: use of computers, position statement*, UKCC, 1992
(8) *Complementary therapies, position statement*, UKCC, 1995
(9) *Acquired Immune Deficiency Syndrome and Human Immune Deficiency Virus Infection (AIDS and HIV Infection)*, UKCC, 1994
(10) *Anonymous Testing for the Prevalence of the Human Immune Deficiency Virus (HIV)*, UKCC, 1994

These documents are available on written request from the Distribution Department at the UKCC.

Laws relevant to these guidelines

(1) Nurses, Midwives and Health Visitors Acts 1979 and 1992
(2) Access to Health Records Act 1990
(3) Family Law Reform Act 1969
(4) Age of Legal Capacity (Scotland) Act 1991
(5) Children Act 1989
(6) Mental Health (Northern Ireland) Order 1986
(7) Mental Health (England and Wales) Act 1983
(8) Mental Health (Scotland) Act 1984
(9) Abortion Act 1967
(10) Human Fertilisation and Embryology Act 1990
(11) Data Protection Act 1984
(12) Access Modification (Health) Order 1987
(13) Computer Misuse Act 1990
(14) European Community Directive 91/507/EEC

These are available from your local branch of Her Majesty's Stationery Office (HMSO).

Appendix 3

Standards for the Administration of Medicines

Introduction

(1) This standards paper replaces the Council's advisory paper *Administration of Medicines* (issued in 1986) [1] and the supplementary circular *The Administration of Medicines* (PC 88/05).[2] The council has prepared this paper to assist practitioners to fulfil the expectations which it has of them, to serve more effectively the interests of patients and clients and to maintain and enhance standards of practice.

(2) The administration of medicines is an important aspect of the professional practice of persons whose names are on the Council's register. It is not solely a mechanistic task to be performed in strict compliance with the written prescription of a medical practitioner. It requires thought and the exercise of professional judgement which is directed to:

(2.1) confirming the correctness of the prescription;
(2.2) judging the suitability of administration at the scheduled time of administration;
(2.3) reinforcing the positive effect of the treatment;
(2.4) enhancing the understanding of patients in respect of their prescribed medication and the avoidance of misuse of these and other medicines; and
(2.5) assisting in assessing the efficacy of medicines and the identification of side effects and interactions.

(3) To meet the standards set out in this paper is to honour, in this aspect of practice, the Council's expectation (set out in the Council's Code of Professional Conduct)[3] that:

'As a registered nurse, midwife or health visitor you are personally accountable for your practice and, in the exercise of your professional accountability, must:

1 act always in such a manner as to promote and safeguard the interests and well-being of patients and clients;
2 ensure that no action or omission on your part, or within your sphere of responsibility, is detrimental to the interests, condition or safety of patients and clients;

3 maintain and improve your professional knowledge and competence;
4 acknowledge any limitations in your knowledge and competence and decline any duties or responsibilities unless able to perform them in a safe and skilled manner;'

(4) This extract from the Code of Professional Conduct applies to all persons on the Council's register irrespective of the part of the register on which their name appears. Although the content of pre-registration education programmes varies, dependent on the part and level of the register involved, the Council expects that, in this area of practice as in all others, all practitioners will have taken steps to develop their knowledge and competence and will have been assisted to this end. The word 'practitioner' is, therefore, used in the remainder of this paper to refer to all registered nurses, midwives and health visitors, each of whom must recognise the personal professional accountability which they bear for their actions. The Council therefore imposes no arbitrary boundaries between the role of the first level and second level registered practitioner in this respect.

Treatment with medicines

(5) The treatment of a patient with medicines for therapeutic, diagnostic or preventative purposes is a process which involves prescribing, dispensing, administering, receiving and recording. The word 'patient' is used for convenience, but implies not only a patient in a hospital or nursing home, but also a resident of a residential home, a client in her or his own home or in a community home, a person attending a clinic or a general practitioner's surgery and an employee attending a workplace occupational health department. 'Patient' refers to the person receiving a prescribed medicine. Each medicine has a product licence, which means that authority has been given to a manufacturer to market a particular product for administration in a particular dosage range and by specified routes.

Prescription

(6) The practitioner administering a medicine against a prescription written by a registered medical practitioner, like the pharmacist responsible for dispensing it, can reasonably expect that the prescription satisfies the following criteria:

(6.1) that it is based, whenever possible, on the patient's awareness of the purpose of the treatment and consent (commonly implicit);
(6.2) that the prescription is either clearly written, typed or computer-generated, and that the entry is indelible and dated;
(6.3) that, where the new prescription replaces an earlier prescription, the latter has been cancelled clearly and the cancellation signed and dated by an authorised registered medical practitioner;
(6.4) that, where a prescribed substance (which replaces an earlier prescription) has been provided for a person residing at home or in a

residential care home and who is dependent on others to assist with the administration, information about the change has been properly communicated;

(6.5) that the prescription provides clear and unequivocal identification of the patient for whom the medicine is intended;

(6.6) that the substance to be administered is clearly specified and, where appropriate, its form (for example tablet, capsule, suppository) stated, together with the strength, dosage, timing and frequency of administration and route of administration;

(6.7) that, where the prescription is provided in an out-patients or community setting, it states the duration of the course before review;

(6.8) that, in the case of controlled drugs, the dosage is written, together with the number of dosage units or total course if in an out-patient or community setting, the whole being in the prescriber's own handwriting;

(6.9) that all other prescriptions will, as a minimum, have been signed by the prescribing doctor and dated;

(6.10) that the registered medical practitioner understands that the administration of medicines on verbal instructions, whether she or he is present or absent, other than in exceptional circumstances, is not acceptable unless covered by the protocol method referred to in paragraph 6.11;

(6.11) that it is understood that, unless provided for in a specific protocol, instruction by telephone to a practitioner to administer a previously unprescribed substance is not acceptable, the use of facsimile transmission (fax) being the preferred method in exceptional circumstances or isolated locations; and

(6.12) that, where it is the wish of the professional staff concerned that practitioners in a particular setting be authorised to administer, on their own authority, certain medicines, a local protocol has been agreed between medical practitioners, nurses and midwives and the pharmacist.

Dispensing

(7) The practitioner administering a medicine dispensed by a pharmacist in response to a medical prescription can reasonably expect that:

(7.1) the pharmacist has checked that the prescription is written correctly so as to avoid misunderstanding or error and is signed by an authorised prescriber;

(7.2) the pharmacist is satisfied that any newly-prescribed medicines will not dangerously interact with or nullify each other;

(7.3) the pharmacist has provided the medicine in a form relevant for administration to the particular patient, provided it in an appropriate container giving the relevant information and advised appropriately on storage and security conditions;

(7.4) where the substance is prescribed in a dose or to be administered by a route which falls outside its product licence, unless to be administered from a stock supply, the pharmacist will have taken steps to ensure that the prescriber is aware and has chosen to exceed that licence;

(7.5) where the prescription for a specific item falls outside the terms of the product licence, whether as to its route of administration, the dosage or some other key factor, the pharmacist will have ensured that the prescriber is aware of this fact and, mindful of her or his accountability in the matter, has made a record on the prescription to this effect and has agreed to dispense the medicine ordered;

(7.6) if the prescription bears any written amendments made and signed by the pharmacist, the prescriber has been consulted and advised and the amendments have been accepted; and

(7.7) the pharmacist, in pursuit of her or his role in monitoring the adverse side-effects of medicines, wishes to be sent any information that the administering practitioner deems relevant.

Standards for the administration of medicines

(8) Notwithstanding the expected adherence by registered medical practitioners and pharmacists to the criteria set out in paragraphs 6 and 7 of this paper, the nurse, midwife or health visitor must, in administering any medicines, in assisting with administration or overseeing any self-administration of medicines, exercise professional judgement and apply knowledge and skill to the situation that pertains at the time.

(9) This means that, as a matter of basic principle, whether administering a medicine, assisting in its administration or overseeing self-administration, the practitioner will be satisfied that she or he:

(9.1) has an understanding of substances used for therapeutic purposes;

(9.2) is able to justify any actions taken; and

(9.3) is prepared to be accountable for the action taken.

(10) Against this background, the practitioner, acting in the interests of the patients, will:

(10.1) be certain of the identity of the patient to whom the medicine is to be administered;

(10.2) ensure that she or he is aware of the patient's current assessment and planned programme of care;

(10.3) pay due regard to the environment in which that care is being given;

(10.4) scrutinise carefully, in the interests of safety, the prescription, where available, and the information provided on the relevant containers;

(10.5) question the medical practitioner or pharmacist, as appropriate, if the prescription or container information is illegible, unclear, ambiguous or incomplete or where it is believed that the dosage or route of administration falls outside the product licence for the particular substance and, where believed necessary, refuse to administer the prescribed substance;

(10.6) refuse to prepare substances for injection in advance of their immediate use and refuse to administer a medicine not placed in a container or drawn into a syringe by her or him, in her or his presence, or prepared by a pharmacist, except in the specific circumstances described in paragraph 40 of this paper and others where similar issues arise; and

(10.7) draw the attention of patients, as appropriate, to patient information leaflets concerning their prescribed medicines.

(11) In addition, acting in the interests of the patient, the practitioner will:

(11.1) check the expiry date of any medicine, if on the container;

(11.2) carefully consider the dosage, method of administration, route and timing of administration in the context of the condition of the specific patient at the operative time;

(11.3) carefully consider whether any of the prescribed medicines will or may dangerously interact with each other;

(11.4) determine whether it is necessary or advisable to withhold the medicine pending consultation with the prescribing medical practitioner, the pharmacist or a fellow professional colleague;

(11.5) contact the prescriber without delay where contra-indications to the administration of any prescribed medicine are observed, first taking the advice of the pharmacist where considered appropriate;

(11.6) make clear, accurate and contemporaneous record of the administration of all medicines administered or deliberately withheld, ensuring that any written entries and the signature are clear and legible;

(11.7) where a medicine is refused by the patient, or the parent refuses to administer or allow administration of that medicine, make a clear and accurate record of the fact without delay, consider whether the refusal of that medicine compromises the patient's condition or the effect of other medicines, assess the situation and contact the prescriber;

(11.8) use the opportunity which administration of a medicine provides for emphasising, to patients and their carers, the importance and implications of the prescribed treatment and for enhancing their understanding of its effects and side-effects;

(11.9) record the positive and negative effects of the medicine and make them known to the prescribing medical practitioner and the pharmacist; and

(11.10) take all possible steps to ensure that replaced prescription entries are correctly deleted to avoid duplication of medicines.

Applying the Standards in a range of settings

Who can administer medicines?

(12) There is a wide spectrum of situations in which medicines are administered ranging, at one extreme, from the patient in an intensive therapy unit who is totally dependent on registered professional staff for her or his care to, at the other extreme, the person in her or his own home administering her or his own

medicines or being assisted in this respect by a relative or another person. The answer to the question of who can administer a medicine must largely depend on where within that spectrum the recipient of the medicines lies.

Administration in the hospital setting

(13) It is the Council's position that, at or near the first stated end of that spectrum, assessment of response to treatment and speedy recognition of contra-indications and side-effects are of great importance. Therefore prescribed medicines should only be administered by registered practitioners who are competent for the purpose and aware of their personal accountability.

(14) In this context it is the Council's position that, in the majority of circumstances, a first level registered nurse, a midwife, or a second level nurse, each of whom has demonstrated the necessary knowledge and competence, should be able to administer medicines without involving a second person. Exceptions to this might be:

- (14.1) where the practitioner is instructing a student;
- (14.2) where the patient's condition makes it necessary; and
- (14.3) where local circumstances make the involvement of two persons desirable in the interests of the patients (for example, in areas of specialist care, such as a paediatric unit without sufficient specialist paediatric nurses or in other acute units dependent on temporary agency or other locum staff).

(15) In respect of the administration of intravenous drugs by practitioners, it is the Council's position that this is acceptable, provided that, as in all other aspects of practice, the practitioner is satisfied with her or his competence and mindful of her or his personal accountability.

(16) The Council is opposed to the involvement of persons who are not registered practitioners in the administration of medicines in acute care settings and with ill or dependent patients, since the requirements of paragraphs 8 to 11 inclusive of this paper cannot then be satisfied. It accepts, however, that the professional judgement of an individual practitioner should be used to identify those situations in which informal carers might be instructed and prepared to accept a delegated responsibility in this respect.

Administration in the domestic or quasi-domestic setting

(17) It is evident that in this setting, on the majority of occasions, there is no involvement of registered practitioners. Where a practitioner engaged in community practice does become involved in assisting with or overseeing administration, then she or he must observe paragraphs 8 to 11 of this paper and apply them to the required degree. She or he must also recognise that, even if not employed in posts requiring registration with the Council, she or he remains accountable to the Council.

(18) The same principles apply where prescribed medicines are being administered to residents in small community homes or in residential care homes. To the

maximum degree possible, though related to their ability to manage the care and administration of their prescribed medicines and comprehend their significance, the residents should be regarded as if in their own home. Where assistance is required, the person providing it fills the role of an informal carer, family member or friend. However, as with the situation described in paragraph 17, where a professional practitioner is involved, a personal accountability is borne. The advice of a community pharmacist should be sought when necessary.

Self-administration of medicines in hospitals or registered nursing homes

(19) The Council welcomes and supports the development of self-administration of medicines and administration by parents to children wherever it is appropriate and the necessary security and storage arrangements are available.

(20) For the hospital patient approaching discharge, but who will continue on a prescribed medicines regime following the return home, there are obvious benefits in adjusting to the responsibility of self-administration while still having access to professional support. It is accepted that, to facilitate this transition, practitioners may assist patients to administer their medicines safely by preparing a form of medication card containing information transcribed from other sources.

(21) For the long stay patient, whether in hospital or a nursing home, self-administration can help foster a feeling of independence and control in one aspect of life.

(22) It is essential, however, that where self-administration is introduced for all or some patients, arrangements must be in place for the appropriate, safe and secure storage of the medicines, access to which is limited to the specific patient.

The use of monitored dosage systems

(23) Monitored dosage systems, for the purpose of this paper, are systems which involve a community pharmacist, in response to the full prescription of medicines for a specific person, dispensing those medicines into a special container with sections for days of the week and times within those days and delivering the container, or supplying the medicines in a special container of blister packs, with appropriate additional information, to the nursing home, residential care home or domestic residence. The Council is aware of the development of such monitored dosage systems and accepts that, provided they are able to satisfy strict criteria established by the Royal Pharmaceutical Society of Great Britain and other official pharmaceutical organisations, that substances which react to each other are not supplied in this way and that they are suitable for the intended purpose as judged by the nursing profession, they have a valuable place in the administration of medicines.

(24) While, to the present, their use has been primarily in registered nursing homes and some community or residential care homes, there seems no reason why, provided the systems can satisfy the standards referred to in paragraph 25, their use should not be extended.

(25) In order to be acceptable for use in hospitals or registered nursing homes, the containers for the medicines must:

(25.1) satisfy the requirements of the Royal Pharmaceutical Society of Great Britain for an original container;
(25.2) be filled by a pharmacist and sealed by her or him or under her or his control and delivered complete to the user;
(25.3) be accompanied by clear and comprehensive documentation which forms the medical practitioner's prescription;
(25.4) bear the means of identifying tablets of similar appearance so that, should it be necessary to withhold one tablet (for example Digoxin), it can be identified from those in the container space for the particular time and day;
(25.5) be able to be stored in a secure place; and
(25.6) make it apparent if the containers (be they blister packs or spaces within a container) have been tampered with between the closure and sealing by the pharmacist and the time of administration.

(26) While the introduction of a monitored dosage system transfers to the pharmacist the responsibility for being satisfied that the container is filled and sealed correctly so as to comply with the prescription, it does not alter the fact that the practitioner administering the medicines must still consider the appropriateness of each medicine at the time administration falls due. It is not the case, therefore, that the use of a monitored dosage system allows the administration of medicines to be undertaken by unqualified personnel.

(27) It is not acceptable, in lieu of a pharmacist-filled monitored dosage system container, for a practitioner to transfer medicines from their original containers into an unsealed container for administration at a later stage by another person, whether or not that person is a registered practitioner. This is an unsafe practice which carries risks for both practitioner and patient. Similarly it is not acceptable to interfere with a sealed section at any time between its closure by the pharmacist and the scheduled time of administration.

The role of nurses, midwives and health visitors in community practice in the administration of medicines

(28) Any practitioner who, whether as a planned intervention or incidentally, becomes involved in administering a medicine, or assisting with or overseeing such administration, must apply paragraphs 8 to 11 of this paper to the degree to which they are relevant.

(29) Where a practitioner working in the community becomes involved in obtaining prescribed medicines for patients, she or he must recognise her or his responsibility for safe transit and correct delivery.

(30) Community psychiatric nurses whose practice involves them in providing assistance to patients to reduce and eliminate their dependence on addictive drugs should ensure that they are aware of the potential value of short term prescriptions and encourage their use where appropriate in the long term

interests of their clients. They must not resort to holding or carrying prescribed controlled drugs to avoid their misuse by those clients.

(31) Special arrangements and certain exemptions apply to occupational health nurses. These are described in Information Document 11 and the Appendices of *A Guide to an Occupational Health Nursing Service; A Handbook for Employers and Nurses*; published by the Royal College of Nursing.[4]

(32) Some practitioners employed in the community, including in particular community nurses, practice nurses and health visitors, in order to enhance disease prevention, will receive requests to participate in vaccination and immunisation programmes. Normally these requests will be accompanied by specific named prescriptions or be covered by a protocol setting out the arrangements within which substances can be administered to certain categories of persons who meet the stated criteria. The facility provided by the Medicines Act 1968[5] for substances to be administered to a number of people in response to an advance 'direction' is valuable in this respect. Where it has not been possible to anticipate the possible need for preventive treatment and there is no relevant protocol or advance direction, particularly in respect of patients about to travel abroad and requiring preventive treatment, a telephone conversation with a registered medical practitioner will suffice as authorisation for a single administration. It is not, however, sufficient as a basis for supplying a quantity of medicines.

Midwives and midwifery practice

(33) Midwives should refer to the current editions of both the Council's *Midwives Rules*[6] and *A Midwife's Code of Practice*[7] and specifically to the sections concerning administration of medicines. At the time of publication of this paper, *Midwives Rules* sets out the practising midwife's responsibility in respect of the administration of medicines and other forms of pain relief. *A Midwife's Code of Practice* refers to the authority provided by the Medicines Act 1968 and the Misuse of Drugs Act 1971,[8] and regulations made as a result, for midwives to obtain and administer certain substances.

What if the Council's standards in paragraphs 8 to 11 cannot be applied?

(34) There are certain situations in which practitioners are involved in the administration of medicines where some of the criteria stated above either cannot be applied or, if applied, would introduce dangerous delay with consequent risk to patients. These will include occupational health settings in some industries, small hospitals with no resident medical staff and possibly some specialist units within larger hospitals and some community settings.

(35) With the exception of the administration of substances for the purpose of vaccination or immunisation described in paragraph 32 above, in any situation in which a practitioner may be expected or required to administer 'prescription-

only medicines' which have not been directly prescribed for a named patient by a registered medical practitioner who has examined the patient and made a diagnosis, it is essential that a clear local policy be determined and made known to all practitioners involved with prescribing and administration. This will make it possible for action to be taken in patients' interests while protecting practitioners from the risk of complaint which might otherwise jeopardise their position.

(36) Therefore, where such a situation will, or may apply, a local policy should be agreed and documented which:

(36.1) states the circumstances in which particular 'prescription-only medicines' may be administered in advance of examination by a doctor;
(36.2) ensures the relevant knowledge and skill of those to be involved in administration;
(36.3) describes the form, route and dosage range of the medicines so authorised; and
(36.4) wherever possible, satisfies the requirements of Section 58 of the Medicines Act 1968 as a 'direction'.

Substances for topical application

(37) The standards set out in this paper apply, to the degree to which they are relevant, to substances used for wound dressing and other topical applications. Where a practitioner uses a substance or product which has not been prescribed, she or he must have considered the matter sufficiently to be able to justify its use in the particular circumstances.

The administration of homoeopathic or herbal substances

(38) Homoeopathic and herbal medicines are subject to the licensing provisions of the Medicines Act 1968, although those on the market when that Act became operative (which means most of those now available) received product licences without any evaluation of their efficacy, safety or quality. Practitioners should, therefore, make themselves generally aware of common substances used in their particular area of practice. It is necessary to respect the right of individuals to administer to themselves, or to request a practitioner to assist in the administration of substances in these categories. If, when faced with a patient or client whose desire to receive medicines of this kind appears to create potential difficulties, or if it is felt that the substances might either be an inappropriate response to the presenting symptoms or likely to negate or enhance the effect of prescribed medicines, the practitioner, acting in the interests of the patient or client, should consider contacting the relevant registered medical practitioner, but must also be mindful of the need not to override the patient's rights.

Complementary and alternative therapies

(39) Some registered nurses, midwives and health visitors, having first undertaken successfully a training in complementary or alternative therapy which involves the use of substances such as essential oils, apply their specialist knowledge and skill in their practice. It is essential that practice in these respects, as in all others, is based upon sound principles, available knowledge and skill. The importance of consent to the use of such treatment must be recognised. So, too, must the practitioner's personal accountability for her or his professional practice.

Practitioners assuming responsibility for care which includes medicines being administered which were previously checked by other practitioners

(40) Paragraph 10.6 of this paper referred to the unacceptability of a practitioner administering a substance drawn into a syringe or container by another practitioner when the practitioner taking over responsibility for the patient was not present. An exception to this is an already established intravenous infusion, the use of a syringe pump or some other kind of continuous or intermittent infusion or injection apparatus, where a valid prescription exists, a responsible practitioner has signed for the container of fluid and any additives being administered and the container is clearly and indelibly labelled. The label must clearly show the contents and be signed and dated. The same measures must apply equally to other means of administration of such substances through, for example, central venous, arterial or epidural lines. Strict discipline must be applied to the recording of any substances being administered by any of the methods referred to in this paragraph and to reporting procedures between staff as they change and transfer responsibility for care.

Management of errors or incidents in the administration of medicines

(41) In a number of its Annual Reports, the Council has recorded its concern that practitioners who have made mistakes under pressure of work, and have been honest and open about those mistakes to their senior staff, appear often to have been made the subject of disciplinary action in a way which seems likely to discourage the reporting of incidents and therefore be to the potential detriment of patients and of standards.

(42) When considering allegations of misconduct arising out of errors in the administration of medicines, the Council's Professional Conduct Committee takes great care to distinguish between those cases where the error was the result of reckless practice and was concealed and those which resulted from serious pressure of work and where there was immediate, honest disclosure in the patient's interest. The Council recognises the prerogative of managers to take

local disciplinary action where it is considered to be appropriate but urges that they also consider each incident in its particular context and similarly discriminate between the two categories described.

(43) The Council's position is that all errors and incidents require a thorough and careful investigation which takes full account of the circumstances and context of the event and the position of the practitioner involved. Events of this kind call equally for sensitive management and a comprehensive assessment of all of the circumstances before a professional and managerial decision is reached on the appropriate way to proceed.

Future arrangements for prescribing by nurses

(44) In March 1992 the Act of Parliament entitled the Medicinal Products: Prescription by Nurses etc Act 1992[9] became law. This legislation is to come into operation in October 1993. The legislation will permit nurses with a district nursing or health visiting qualification to prescribe certain products from a Nurse Prescribers' Formulary. The statutory rules, yet to be completed, will specify the categories of nurses who can prescribe under this limited legislation. The Council will issue further information concerning this important new legislation prior to it becoming operative.

(45) Enquiries in respect of this Council paper should be directed to the:

Registrar and Chief Executive
United Kingdom Central Council
for Nursing, Midwifery and
Health Visiting
23 Portland Place
London W1N 3AF

References

1 United Kingdom Central Council for Nursing, Midwifery and Health Visiting, *Administration of Medicines; A UKCC Advisory Paper; A framework to assist individual professional judgement and the development of local policies and guidelines*, April 1986.

2 United Kingdom Central Council for Nursing, Midwifery and Health Visiting, *The Administration of Medicines*, PC 88/05, September 1988.

3 United Kingdom Central Council for Nursing, Midwifery and Health Visiting, *Code of Professional Conduct for the Nurse, Midwife and Health Visitor*, Third Edition, June 1992.

4 Royal College of Nursing, *A Guide to an Occupational Health Nursing Service; A Handbook for Employers and Nurses*, Second Edition 1991.

5 Medicines Act 1968, Her Majesty's Stationery Office, London, Reprinted 1986.

6 United Kingdom Central Council for Nursing, Midwifery and Health Visiting, *Midwives Rules*, March 1991.

7 United Kingdom Central Council for Nursing, Midwifery and Health Visiting, *A Midwife's Code of Practice*, March 1991.

8 Misuse of Drugs Act 1971, Her Majesty's Stationery Office, London, Reprinted 1985.

9 *Medicinal Products: Prescription by Nurses etc Act 1992*, Her Majesty's Stationery Office, London, 1992.

Appendix 4

Standards for Records and Record Keeping

Introduction

(1) The important activity of making and keeping records is an essential and integral part of care and not a distraction from its provision. There is, however, substantial evidence to indicate that inadequate and inappropriate record keeping concerning the care of patients and clients neglects their interests through:

(1.1) impairing continuity of care;
(1.2) introducing discontinuity of communication between staff;
(1.3) creating the risk of medication or other treatment being duplicated or omitted;
(1.4) failing to focus attention on early signs of deviation from the norm; and
(1.5) failing to place on record significant observations and conclusions.

(2) For these reasons the Council has prepared this standards paper to assist its practitioners to fulfil the expectations it has of them and to serve more effectively the interests of their patients and clients.

(3) To meet the standards set out in this document is to honour, in this aspect of practice, the Council's expectation (set out in the Code of Professional Conduct for the Nurse, Midwife and Health Visitor)[1] that:

> 'As a registered nurse, midwife or health visitor you are personally accountable for your practice and, in the exercise of your professional accountability, must:
>
> 1 act always in such a manner as to promote and safeguard the interests and well-being of patients and clients;
>
> 2 ensure that no action or omission on your part, or within your sphere of responsibility, is detrimental to the interests, condition or safety of patients and clients;'

The purpose of records

(4) The purpose of records created and maintained by registered nurses, midwives and health visitors is to:

(4.1) provide accurate, current, comprehensive and concise information concerning the condition and care of the patient or client and associated observations;

(4.2) provide a record of any problems that arise and the action taken in response to them;

(4.3) provide evidence of care required, intervention by professional practitioners and patient or client responses;

(4.4) include a record of any factors (physical, psychological or social) that appear to affect the patient or client;

(4.5) record the chronology of events and the reasons for any decisions made;

(4.6) support standard setting, quality assessment and audit; and

(4.7) provide a baseline record against which improvement or deterioration may be judged.

The importance of records

(5) Effective record keeping by nurses, midwives and health visitors is a means of:

(5.1) communicating with others and describing what has been observed or done;

(5.2) identifying the discrete role played by nurses, midwives and health visitors in care;

(5.3) organising communication and the dissemination of information among the members of the team providing care for a patient or client;

(5.4) demonstrating the chronology of events, the factors observed and the response to care and treatment and

(5.5) demonstrating the properly considered clinical decisions relating to patient care.

Standards for records – key features

(6) In addition to fulfilling the purposes set out in paragraph 4, properly made and maintained records will:

(6.1) be made as soon as possible after the events to which they relate;

(6.2) identify factors which jeopardise standards or place the patient or client at risk;

(6.3) provide evidence of the need, in specific cases, for practitioners with special knowledge and skills;

(6.4) aid patient or client involvement in their own care;

(6.5) provide 'protection' for staff against any future complaint which may be made; and

(6.6) be written, wherever possible, in terms which the patient or client will be able to understand.

Standards for records – ethical aspects

(7) A correctly made record honours the ethical concepts on which good practice is based and demonstrates the basis of the professional and clinical decisions made.

(8) A basic tenet of records and record keeping is that those who make, access and use the records understand the ethical concepts of professional practice which relate to them. These will include, in particular, the need to protect confidentiality, to ensure true consent and to assist patients and clients to make informed decisions.

(9) The originator will ensure that the entry in a record that she or he makes is totally accurate and based on respect for truth and integrity.

Standards for records – recording decisions on resuscitation

(10) It is essential that the records on the subject of resuscitation accurately and explicitly reflect any wishes of a patient expressed when legally and mentally competent or those of the patient's next of kin or other significant persons when those circumstances do not apply. This is particularly important when a patient has expressed a wish not to be resuscitated. This is to say that the wishes of a patient, made and expressed when she or he was legally and mentally competent, should be respected.

(11) Where the views of the patient and/or those of 'significant others' in relationship to them have not been recorded, but a decision not to resuscitate has been made on clinical grounds by the relevant medical staff, this also should be entered in writing in the medical record and the entry must be signed and dated by the responsible registered medical practitioner. Wherever possible this should be a team decision which, though made by the medical staff, would take the informed views of the nursing staff (and, where applicable, midwifery staff) into account. The patient's family or other significant personal carers should, wherever possible, be consulted.

(12) Whether the circumstances in paragraph 10 or paragraph 11 apply, the entry must be able to be located easily and quickly in the medical record and must include a time limit for which it is to apply before review. Nursing and midwifery staff must not enter this decision in the nursing or midwifery record unless it has first been entered in the medical record in the way described in paragraph 11 above.

Standards for records – essential elements

(13) In order to fulfil the purpose stated in paragraph 4, to be effective and to meet the standards set out above, records must:

(13.1) be written legibly and indelibly;
(13.2) be clear and unambiguous;

(13.3) be accurate in each entry as to date and time;

(13.4) ensure that alterations are made by scoring out with a single line followed by the initialled, dated and timed correct entry;

(13.5) ensure that additions to existing entries are individually dated, timed and signed;

(13.6) not include abbreviations, meaningless phrases and offensive subjective statements unrelated to the patient's care and associated observations;

(13.7) not allow the use of initials for major entries and, where their use is allowed for other entries, ensure that local arrangements for identifying initials and signatures exist; and

(13.8) not include entries made in pencil or blue ink, the former carrying the risk of erasure and the latter (where photocopying is required) of poor quality reproduction.

(14) In summary, the record:

(14.1) is directed primarily to serving the interests and care of the patient or client to whom the record relates and enabling the provision of care, the prevention of disease and the promotion of health and

(14.2) will demonstrate the chronology of events and all significant consultations, assessments, observations, decisions, interventions and outcomes.

(15) In hospitals or other institutions providing care, a local index record of signatures should be held. Where initials are regarded as acceptable for any purpose, these also should feature in the index, together with the full name in printed form.

The 'process approach' or 'planned individualised care' approach to nursing and midwifery care

(16) Given the nature of care plans and records associated with the planned individual care approach, this important aspect of records must satisfy the criteria specified in paragraphs 4 to 15 above. The 'process' approach assists a systematic approach to practice. It also provides a framework for the documentation of that practice. The term therefore describes the continuum of distinctly separate yet interrelated activities of practice, assessment, planning, implementation and evaluation of care.

(17) Meticulous and timely documentation provides evidence of the practitioner's actions, the patient's or client's response to those actions and the plans and goals which direct the care of the patient or client.

(18) The preparation and completion of care plans will, therefore, in addition to satisfying the criteria set out in paragraphs 4 to 15 above, demonstrate that each step in what is a continuing process has been followed and provides the basis for further goal setting and actions.

(19) The making of entries will be organised so that:

(19.1) a measurable, up to date, description of the condition of the patient or client and the care delivered can be easily communicated to others and

(19.2) the plan and other records complement each other.

(20) The practitioner, in applying the process and using the plan, will distinguish between those matters which must be recorded in advance (such as planning and goals) and those which can only be current or slightly retrospective (such as observations and evaluation). Equally, the distinction must be made between entries on papers, (for example, planning forms) which may not be locally retained, and other forms which are part of the clinical nursing or midwifery care records which record changes and events and must be retained.

The legal status of records and its implications

(21) Any document which records any aspect of the care of a patient or client can be required as evidence before a court of law or before the Preliminary Proceedings Committee or Professional Conduct Committee of the Council (the UKCC) or other similar regulatory bodies for the health care professions including the General Medical Council, the comparable body to the UKCC for the medical profession.

(22) For this, in addition to their primary purpose of serving the interests of the patient or client, the records should provide:

(22.1) a comprehensive picture of care delivered, associated outcomes and other relevant information;
(22.2) pertinent information about the condition of the patient or client at any given time and the measures taken to respond to identified need;
(22.3) evidence that the practitioner's common law duty of care has been understood and honoured and
(22.4) a record of the arrangements made for continuity of a patient's care on discharge from hospital.

(23) Particular care will be exercised and frequent record entries made where patients or clients present complex problems, show deviation from the norm, require more intensive care than normal, are confused and disoriented or in other ways give cause for concern.

(24) In situations where the condition of the patient or client is apparently unchanging, local agreement will be necessary in respect of the maximum time allowed to elapse between entries in patient or client records and the nature of those entries. All exceptional events, however, must be recorded and the Council will expect nurses, midwives and health visitors to exercise suitable judgement about entries in the record.

(25) Ownership of the contents of a record would normally be seen as residing with the originator of any particular entry. In practice, however, where the professional practitioner is a salaried employee of the health services, the question of ownership turns on ownership of the document on which the record is made. Ownership does not rest with the patient or client, as the creation of law to grant patient or client access in certain circumstances clearly reveals.

(26) Midwives must ensure that they are aware of and comply with the requirements in respect of records set out in the Council's *Midwives Rules*.

(27) It is essential that members of the professions must be involved in local discussions to determine policies concerning the retention or disposal of all or any part of records which they or their colleagues make. Such policies must be determined with recognition of any aspects of law affecting the duration of retention and make explicit the period for which specific categories of records are to be retained. Any documents which form part of the chronological clinical care record should be retained.

Retention of obstetric records

(28) All essential obstetric records (such as those recording the care of a mother and baby during pregnancy, labour and the puerperium, including all test results, prescription forms and records of medicines administered) must be retained. Decisions concerning those records which are to be regarded as essential must not be made at local level without involving senior medical practitioners concerned with the provision of maternity and neo-natal services and a senior practising midwife.

(29) Those involved in determining policy at local level must ensure that the records retained are comprehensive (in that they include both hospital, community midwifery records and those held by mothers during pregnancy and the puerperium) and are such as to facilitate any investigations required as a result of action brought under the Congenital Disabilities (Civil Liabilities) Act 1976 or any other litigation.

Patient or client held records

(30) The Council is in favour of patients and clients being given custody of their own health care records in circumstances where it is appropriate. Patient or client held records help to emphasise and make clear the practitioner's responsibility to the patient or client by sharing any information held or assessments made and illustrate the involvement of the patient or client in their own care.

(31) Evidence from those places where this has become the practice indicates that there are no substantial drawbacks and considerable ethical benefits to be derived from patients or clients having custody of their records. This immediately disposes of any difficulties concerning access and reinforces the discipline that should apply to making entries in records.

(32) A small number of instances will inevitably arise, where a system of patient or client held records is in operation, in which the health professional concerned will feel that her or his particular concerns or anxieties (for example about the possibility of child abuse) require that a supplementary record be created and held by the practitioner. To make and keep such a record can, in appropriate circumstances, be regarded as good practice. It should be the exception rather than the norm, however, and should not extend to keeping full duplicate records unless in the most unusual circumstances.

Patient or client access to records

(33) With effect from 1 November 1991, patients and clients have had the right of access to manual records about themselves made from that date as a result of the Access to Health Records Act 1990 coming into effect. This has brought such records into line with computer held records which have been required to be accessible to patients since the Data Protection Act 1984 became operative.

(34) These Acts give the right of access, but the health professional most directly concerned (which, in certain cases will be the nurse, midwife or health visitor) is permitted to withhold information which she or he believes might cause serious harm to the physical or mental health of the patient or client or which would identify a third party. The system for dealing with applications for access is explained in the *Access to Health Records Act 1990: a Guide for the NHS*, published by the Government Health Departments.[2]

(35) The Council fully supports the principle of open access to records contained in these Acts, and the guidance notes concerning their operation, and trusts that access will not be unreasonably denied or limited.

(36) All practitioners who create records or make entries in any records must be aware of the rights of the patient or client in this regard, give careful consideration to the language and terminology employed and recognise the positive advantages of greater trust and confidence of patients and clients in the professions that can result from this development.

Shared records

(37) The Council recognises the advantages of 'shared' records in which all health professionals involved in the care and treatment of an individual make entries in a single record and in accordance with a broadly agreed local protocol. These are seen as particularly valuable in midwifery practice. The Council supports this practice where circumstances lend themselves to it and where relevant preparatory work has been undertaken. Each practitioner's contribution to such records should be seen as of equal importance. This reflects the collaborative and cooperative working within the health care team on which emphasis is laid by the Council in its Code of Professional Conduct for the Nurse, Midwife and Health Visitor. The same right of access to records by the patient or client exists where a system of shared records is in use. It is essential, therefore, that local agreement is reached to identify the lead professional to be responsible for considering requests from patients and clients for access in particular circumstances.

Computer held records

(38) The application of computer technology should not be allowed to breach the important principle of confidentiality. To say this is not to oppose the use of computer held records, whether specific to one profession or shared between

professions. Practitioners must satisfy themselves about the security of the system used and ascertain which categories of staff have access to the records to which they are expected to contribute important, personal and confidential information.

(39) Where computer technology is employed it must provide a means of maintaining or enhancing service to patients or clients and avoid the risk of inadvertent breaches of confidentiality. It must not impose a limit on the amount of text a practitioner may enter if the consequence is that it impedes the compilation of a sufficiently comprehensive record. The case for it has to be considered in association with the questions of access, patient or client held records, shared records and audit. Local protocols must include means of authenticating an entry in the absence of a written signature and must indicate clearly the identity of the originator of that entry.

The practitioner's accountability for entries made by others

(40) Irrespective of the type of record or the form or medium employed to create and access it, the registered nurse, midwife or health visitor must recognise her or his personal accountability for entries to records made by students or others under their supervision.

Summary of the principles underpinning records and record keeping

(41) The following principles must apply:

(41.1) the record is directed primarily to serving the interests of the patient or client to whom it relates and enabling the provision of care, the prevention of disease and the promotion of health;
(41.2) the record demonstrates the accurate chronology of events and all significant consultations, assessments, observations, decisions, interventions and outcomes;
(41.3) the record and the activity of record keeping is an integral and essential part of care and not a distraction from its provision;
(41.4) the record is clear and unambiguous;
(41.5) the record contains entries recording facts and observations written at the time of, or soon after, the events described;
(41.6) the record provides a safe and effective means of communication between members of the health care team and supports continuity of care;
(41.7) the record demonstrates that the practitioner's duty of care has been fulfilled;
(41.8) the systems for record keeping exclude unauthorised access and breaches of confidentiality; and
(41.9) the record is constructed and completed in such a manner as to facilitate the monitoring of standards, audit, quality assurance and the investigation of complaints.

(42) Enquiries in respect of this Council paper should be directed to the:

Registrar and Chief Executive
United Kingdom Central Council
for Nursing, Midwifery and
Health Visiting
23 Portland Place
London
W1N 3AF

References

1 *Code of Professional Conduct for the Nurse, Midwife and Health Visitor*; UKCC, London, 1992.

2 *Access to Health Records Act 1990: a Guide for the NHS*; Government Health Departments, 1990.

Appendix 5

The Scope of Professional Practice
A UKCC Position Statement

Introduction

(1) The practice of nursing, midwifery and health visiting requires the application of knowledge and the simultaneous exercise of judgement and skill. Practice takes place in a context of continuing change and development. Such change and development may result from advances in research leading to improvements in treatment and care, from alterations to the provision of health and social care services, as a result of changes in local policies and as a result of new approaches to professional practice. Practice must, therefore, be sensitive, relevant and responsive to the needs of individual patients and clients and have the capacity to adjust, where and when appropriate, to changing circumstances.

(2) Education and experience form the foundation on which nurses, midwives and health visitors exercise judgement and skill, these, naturally, being developed and refined over time. The range of responsibilities which fall to individual nurses, midwives and health visitors should be related to their personal experience, education and skill. This range of responsibilities is described here as the 'scope of professional practice' and this paper sets out the Council's principles on which any adjustment to the scope of professional practice should be based.

Education for professional practice

(3) Just as practice must remain dynamic, sensitive, relevant and responsive to the changing needs of patients and clients, so too must education for practice. Pre-registration education prepares nurses, midwives and health visitors for safe practice at the point of registration. The pre-registration curriculum will continue to change over time to absorb relevant changes in care as advances are made. Pre-registration education is, therefore, a foundation for professional practice and a means of equipping nurses, midwives and health visitors with the necessary knowledge and skills to assume responsibility as registered practitioners. This foundation education alone, however, cannot effectively meet the changing and complex demands of the range of modern health care. Post-registration education equips practitioners with additional and more specialist

skills necessary to meet the special needs of patients and clients. There is a broad range of post-registration provision and the Council regards adequate and effective provision of quality education as a pre-requisite of quality care.

Registration and the Code of Professional Conduct for the nurse, midwife and health visitor

(4) The act of registration by the Council confers on individual nurses, midwives and health visitors the legal right to practise and to use the title 'registered'. From the point of registration, each practitioner is subject to the Council's Code of Professional Conduct and accountable for his or her practice and conduct. The Code provides a statement of the values of the professions and establishes the framework within which practitioners practise and conduct themselves. The act of registration and the expectations stated in the Code are central to the Council's key role in regulating the standards of the professions in the interest of patients and clients and of society as a whole.

(5) Once registered, each nurse, midwife and health visitor remains subject to the Code and ultimately accountable to the Council for his or her actions and omissions. This position applies regardless of the employment circumstances and regardless of whether or not individuals are actively engaged in practice. This position will only change if the decision is made by the Council (through clearly established legal processes related to professional misconduct or unfitness to practise due to illness) to remove a name from the Council's register. This reflects the key, central role which the registration process plays in maintaining standards in the public interest. On the specific question of employment of nurses in the personal social services in general and the residential care sector in particular, the Council recognises that there are ambiguities. These are addressed in paragraphs 20 and 21 of this paper.

The Code of Professional Conduct and the scope of professional practice

(6) The Code includes a number of explicit clauses which relate to changes to the scope of practice in nursing, midwifery and health visiting. These clauses are:

'As a registered nurse, midwife or health visitor you are personally accountable for your practice and, in the exercise of your professional accountability, must:

1 act always in such a manner as to promote and safeguard the interests and well-being of patients and clients;
2 ensure that no action or omission on your part, or within your sphere of responsibility, is detrimental to the interests, condition or safety of patients and clients;
3 maintain and improve your professional knowledge and competence
4 acknowledge any limitations in your knowledge and competence and

decline any duties or responsibilities unless able to perform them in a safe and skilled manner;

(7) The Code, therefore, provides a firm bedrock upon which decisions about adjustments to the scope of professional practice can be made. There are, however, important distinctions relating to the scope of practice in nursing, in midwifery and in health visiting. These are described in the paragraphs that follow the Council's principles for adjusting the scope of practice. These principles apply to the practice of nursing, midwifery and health visiting addressed later in this paper and to any application of complementary or alternative and other therapies by nurses, midwives or health visitors.

Principles for adjusting the scope of practice

(8) Although the practices of nursing, midwifery and health visiting differ widely, the same principles apply to the scope of practice in each of these professions. The following principles are based upon the Council's Code of Professional Conduct and, in particular, on the emphasis which the Code places upon knowledge, skill, responsibility and accountability. The principles which should govern adjustments to the scope of professional practice are those which follow.

(9) The registered nurse, midwife or health visitor:

(9.1) must be satisfied that each aspect of practice is directed to meeting the needs and serving the interests of the patient or client;

(9.2) must endeavour always to achieve, maintain and develop knowledge, skill and competence to respond to those needs and interests;

(9.3) must honestly acknowledge any limits of personal knowledge and skill and take steps to remedy any relevant deficits in order effectively and appropriately to meet the needs of patients and clients;

(9.4) must ensure that any enlargement or adjustment of the scope of personal professional practice must be achieved without compromising or fragmenting existing aspects of professional practice and care and that the requirements of the Council's Code of Professional Conduct are satisfied throughout the whole area of practice;

(9.5) must recognise and honour the direct or indirect personal accountability borne for all aspects of professional practice; and

(9.6) must, in serving the interests of patients and clients and the wider interests of society, avoid any inappropriate delegation to others which compromises those interests.

(10) These principles for practice should enhance trust and confidence within a health care team and promote further the important collaborative work between medical and nursing, midwifery and health visiting practitioners upon which good practice and care depends.

(11) The Council recognises that care by registered nurses, midwives and health visitors is provided in health care, social care and domestic settings. Patients and clients require skilled care from registered practitioners and support staff

require direction and supervision from these same practitioners. These matters are directly concerned with standards of care. This paper, therefore, also addresses the matter of the 'identified' practitioner, practice in the personal social services and residential care sector and support for professional practice.

The scope and 'extended practice' of nursing

(12) The practice of nursing has traditionally been based on the premise that pre-registration education equips the nurse to perform at a certain level and to encompass a particular range of activities. It is also based on the premise that any widening of that range and enhancement of the nurse's practice requires 'official' extension of that role by certification.

(13) The Council considers that the terms 'extended' or 'extending' roles which have been associated with this system are no longer suitable since they limit, rather than extend, the parameters of practice. As a result, many practitioners have been prevented from fulfilling their potential for the benefit of patients. The Council also believes that a concentration on 'activities' can detract from the importance of holistic nursing care. The Council has therefore determined the principles set out in paragraphs 8 to 10 inclusive to provide the basis for ensuring that practice remains dynamic and is able readily and appropriately to adjust to meet changing care needs.

(14) The reality is that the practice of nursing, and education for that practice, will continue to be shaped by developments in care and treatment, and by other events which influence it. This equally applies to midwifery and health visiting. *In order to bring into proper focus the professional responsibility and consequent accountability of individual practitioners, it is the Council's principles for practice rather than certificates for tasks which should form the basis for adjustments to the scope of practice.*

The scope of midwifery practice

(15) The position in relation to midwifery practice is set out in the Council's Midwife's Code of Practice. This indicates that it is the individual midwife's responsibility to maintain and develop the competence which she has acquired during her training, recognising the sphere of practice in which she is deemed to be equipped to practise with safety and competence. It also indicates that, while some developments in midwifery become an essential and integral part of the role of every midwife (and are subsequently incorporated into pre-registration education), other developments may require particular midwives to acquire new skills because of the particular settings in which they are practising. The importance of local policies which are in accord with the Council's policies and standards and the guidelines issued by the National Boards for Nursing, Midwifery and Health Visiting is self-evident. The importance of the midwife practising outside the area of her employing authority or outside the National Health Service discussing the full scope of her practice with her supervisor of midwives is emphasised in the Midwife's Code of Practice.

(16) It can be seen from this position that it is accepted by the Council that some developments in midwifery care can become an integral part of the role of *all* midwives and other developments may become part of the role of some midwives. The Council believes that the Midwife's Code of Practice, cited above, and the Code of Professional Conduct, together provide key principles to underpin the scope of midwifery practice. These are now supplemented by those stated in paragraphs 8 to 10 inclusive of this paper.

The scope of health visiting practice

(17) The position of health visiting differs from that of nursing and midwifery, as there are frequent occasions when the full contribution of health visitors may not find expression where it is most needed. There is, for example, often a concentration on the role of the health visitor in relation to those in the under-five age group at the expense of other groups in the community who need, and would benefit from, the special preparation and skill of health visitors. These circumstances have the effect of constraining practice and limiting the degree to which individuals and communities are able to benefit from the knowledge and skill of health visitors. There is merit in allowing health visitors, where they judge it to be appropriate, to use the full range of their skills in response to needs identified in the pursuit of their health visiting practice. To single out any aspect of practice would be unwise but, where health and nursing need is identified, the health visitor is well placed to determine what intervention may be necessary and able to draw on both her nursing and health visiting education.

(18) The community setting of health visiting practice, the relationship between numerous agencies and services and the health visitor's professional relationship with clients and their families are factors which must be taken into consideration. The health visitor, in all aspects of her practice, is subject to the Council's Code of Professional Conduct and should also satisfy the requirements of paragraphs 8 to 10 inclusive of this paper.

Practice and the 'identified' nurse, midwife and health visitor

(19) The Council recognises that, in a growing number of settings, patients and clients will be in the care of an 'identified' practitioner. The practitioner may be identified as the 'named' practitioner or as the primary, associate or sole practitioner providing nursing, midwifery or health visiting care. In such roles, individuals assume key responsibility for coordinating and supervising the delivery of care, drawing on the general and special resources of colleagues where appropriate. Professional practice naturally involves recognising and accepting accountability for these matters. The Council expects that practitioners will recognise the need to provide all necessary support for colleagues and ensure that practice is underpinned by the required knowledge and skill. The Council equally expects that practitioners identified in one of these ways will be fully prepared for, and supported, in this key role.

Practice in the personal social services and residential care sector

(20) The Council recognises that the community nursing services have a duty to provide a nursing service to those in need of nursing care in the personal social services and residential care sector. Registered nurses who are employed in this sector, whether in homes or in the provision of other services, remain accountable to the Council and subject to the Council's Code of Professional Conduct, even if their posts do not require nursing qualifications. In this regard, as explained in paragraph 5 of this paper, the position of such nurses is the same as that of nurses engaged in direct professional nursing practice.

(21) The Council requires that registered nurses employed in such circumstances will use their judgement and discretion to identify the nursing needs of residents and others for whom they may have responsibility, and will comply with any requirements of the Council. The Council expects that employers will recognise the advantages to the personal social services and residential care sector which result from the employment of registered nurses.

Support for professional practice

(22) Nurses, midwives and health visitors require support in their work. In institutional and community settings, a range of support staff form part of the team. The development of the health care assistant role is linked with a form of vocational training. The Council does not have a direct role in this training, but recognises that this development has an impact upon aspects of care and on the practice and standard of nursing, midwifery and health visiting, for which the Council is responsible.

(23) The Council's position in relation to support roles is as follows:

- (23.1) health care assistants to registered nurses, midwives and health visitors must work under the direction and supervision of those registered practitioners;
- (23.2) registered nurses, midwives and health visitors must remain accountable for assessment, planning and standards of care and for determining the activity of their support staff;
- (23.3) health care assistants must not be allowed to work beyond their level of competence;
- (23.4) continuity of care and appropriate skill/staff mix is important, so health care assistants should be integral members of the caring team;
- (23.5) standards of care must be safeguarded and the need for patients and clients, across the spectrum of health care, to receive skilled professional nursing, midwifery and health visiting assessment and care must be recognised as of primary importance;
- (23.6) health care assistants with the desire and ability to progress to professional education should be encouraged to obtain vocational qualifications, some of which may be approved by the Council as acceptable entry criteria into programmes of professional education; and

(23.7) registered nurses, midwives and health visitors should be involved in these developments so that the support role can be designed to ensure that professional skills are used most appropriately for the benefit of patients and clients.

Conclusion

(24) The principles set out in paragraphs 8 to 10 inclusive of this paper should form the basis for any decisions relating to adjustments to the scope of practice. These principles should replace the system of certification for specific tasks. They provide a realistic, effective and rational approach to adjustments to professional practice.

(25) This change has consequences for managers of clinical practice and professional leaders of nursing, midwifery and health visiting, who must ensure that local policies and procedures are based upon the principles set out in this paper and in the Council's Code of Professional Conduct. Any local arrangements must ensure that registered nurses, midwives and health visitors are assisted to undertake, and are enabled to fulfil, any suitable adjustments to their scope of practice.

(26) This statement sets out the Council's position relating to the scope of professional practice of the professions it regulates, to the 'identified' practitioner, to practice in the residential care sector and to support staff. The Council hopes that this statement, and the principles which it sets out, will provide a clear framework for the logical and desirable development of practice and for the management of practice and care teams. The framework provides for greater flexibility in practice and for enhancing the contribution to care of nurses, midwives and health visitors. Above all, the framework and the principles reflect the personal responsibility and accountability of individual practitioners, entrusted by the Council to protect and improve standards of care.

(27) Enquiries in respect of this Council paper should be directed to the:

Registrar and Chief Executive
United Kingdom Central Council
for Nursing, Midwifery and Health Visiting
23 Portland Place
London
W1N 3AF

Appendix 6

Complaints about Professional Conduct

Preface

The United Kingdom Central Council for Nursing, Midwifery and Health visiting (abbreviated to UKCC and referred to as the Council) is the statutory body responsible for regulating nursing, midwifery and health visiting throughout the United Kingdom. The Council is charged by Parliament with the duty to establish and improve standards of training and professional conduct for nurses, midwives and health visitors. The means of regulation include determining standards for entry to the professions, standards for education, and for conduct. The right to practise is conferred by the Council by registration and this right may be removed only by the Council.

The Statutory Rules of the Council[1] which govern the Council's professional conduct duties state that the term 'misconduct', which forms part of the measure against which allegations are judged, is defined as "conduct unworthy of a registered nurse, midwife, or health visitor . . .".[2] This explanatory paper has been produced to assist those considering submitting either allegations of misconduct against a practitioner whose name appears on the Council's Professional Register or submitting allegations that the fitness to practise of any such practitioner is seriously impaired by illness.[3] The Council hopes that this explanation will be a valuable resource. Further information about the work of the Council may be obtained from the:

Registrar and Chief Executive
UKCC
23 Portland Place
London
W1N 3AF

1 Statutory Instrument 1993 No. 893, The Nurses, Midwives and Health Visitors (Professional Conduct) Rules 1993 Approval Order 1993.

2 Rule 1(2)(k) Statutory Instrument 1993 No. 893, The Nurses, Midwives and Health Visitors (Professional Conduct) Rules 1993 Approval Order 1993.

3 In the text which follows, the use of the female gender equally implies the male.

Introduction

Section 1

(1.1) Section 12 of the Nurses, Midwives and Health Visitors Act 1979, as amended by Section 8 of the Nurses, Midwives and Health Visitors Act 1992, requires the Council to make Statutory Rules (that is, to prepare subordinate law for approval by senior Government law officers) governing the circumstances and the means by which a person's name may be removed from the register.

(1.2) These rules require the Council to:

(1.2.1) set up two Committees drawn from its Members to consider allegations of misconduct, or fitness to practise of registered practitioners and to determine whether the practitioner should be referred for a hearing. Any such Committee is a Preliminary Proceedings Committee or a Professional Screeners Meeting; and

(1.2.2) set up two Committees drawn from its Members to hear evidence of allegations of misconduct or fitness to practise of registered practitioners and to determine whether the practitioner's registration should be suspended or her name removed from the register. Any such Committee is a Professional Conduct Committee or Health Committee.

(1.3) Sections 3 to 7 of this document, together with Annexes A and B, provide a brief explanation of the process of investigation, hearing and judgement of allegations of misconduct. These sections also provide information (based on Professional Conduct Committee decisions during the period 1984–1992) about categories of offence which have often led to removal from the register and those which have not usually resulted in use of that sanction.

(1.4) Sections 8 to 11 of this document, together with Annexe C, provide a brief explanation of the process of assembling medical and other relevant information, consideration by the Panel of Screeners, hearing before the Health Committee and judgement of allegations of unfitness to practise due to illness. It also provides information about categories of illness which often lead to removal from the register.

Legal and professional judgements

Section 2

(2.1) Members of Committees dealing with allegations of misconduct have two principal tasks to undertake before making any judgements about a practitioner's registration status. The first task is to decide whether the facts alleged against a practitioner are proven. The standard of proof required to make this judgement is the equivalent of the criminal burden of proof, which is 'beyond reasonable doubt' or 'satisfied so that you are sure'. The second task is to determine whether the facts proved constitute misconduct. The standard for this judgement was clearly set out by Dame Catherine Hall in 1983, who stated that:

> 'The standard which the Committee takes as its yardstick is not the highest standard which a professional person might attain, but the standard which can reasonably be expected of an average practitioner'.[1]

The Council's expectations of all practitioners are set out in the Council's Code of Professional Conduct.

(2.2) Members of Committees dealing with the question of whether a practitioner's fitness to practise is serioully impaired by reason of ill health have a different task. They will be considering whether, based on medical evidence and their own judgement, a practitioner's fitness to practise is so impaired that she is likely to be a danger to the vulnerable public.

(2.3) However, the purpose of these Committee proceedings is not:

- (2.3.1) to punish the practitioner appearing before the Committee (though the person whose name is removed may so interpret a decision of removal from the register);
- (2.3.2) to provide an employer with grounds to dismiss the practitioner; or
- (2.3.3) to provide an employer with an additional avenue of complaint to use when an appeal against dismissal has been upheld.

Complaints alleging misconduct

Section 3

Who can forward complaints alleging misconduct?

(3.1) It is any person's right to allege that the actions or omissions of a registered nurse, midwife or health visitor constitute misconduct in a professional sense and call into question her continued registration status.

(3.2) This right equally applies to any employee of an organisation providing health care as much as to any other private citizen. Where the employee is a registered nurse, midwife or health visitor, there are circumstances in which that right becomes a duty.

When should a complaint be made?

(3.3) Where the complaint arises from an incident associated with the practitioner's professional practice, which is not and has not been the subject of criminal proceedings, it should be reported as soon as possible. This helps to ensure that the incident will be fresh in the memories of potential witnesses and also that those witnesses will still be readily available. If a matter is serious enough to warrant an allegation of misconduct, it should be reported immediately rather than eventually.

---

1 Extract from the statement made at the first Professional Conduct Committee 21 July 1983, by Dame Catherine Hall, Chairman of the Council.

(3.4) The formal report of a complaint alleging misconduct should not be delayed pending the completion of employment appeal procedures.

(3.5) Many complaints alleging misconduct follow criminal court hearings where guilt has been proved. There are well established systems for a wide range of criminal findings to be reported by the police or the courts.

(3.6) A complaint can be submitted by any person who has knowledge of a court hearing involving a person whose name appears on the Council's register, and who believes that the offences of which the practitioner has been found guilty call into question her future registration status.

How should a complaint alleging misconduct be made?

(3.7) Complaints alleging misconduct should be made in writing to the Council at the address listed at the end of this document. The letter should set out the essential details of the complaint in succinct terms, and provide as much information as is available to assist identification of the practitioner on the Council's register. When the practitioner has been identified, the letter of complaint, or a summary of it, will be sent to the practitioner for comment.

What factors should a potential complainant bear in mind?

(3.8) The points made in paragraph 2.3 of this document are very important.

(3.9) Following investigation, if the case is referred by the Preliminary Proceedings Committee to the Professional Conduct Committee for a hearing, evidence in support of the allegations of misconduct must be given by witnesses testifying under oath in a public hearing.

(3.10) Potential complainants must also note that the standards of evidence and proof required are the same as those applying in criminal courts. 'Hearsay' or 'indirect' evidence is not admissible. Before finding any allegation proven, the Committee Members, having heard evidence in accordance with strict rules, must be satisfied to the degree of being sure. Probability is not enough when the serious sanction of removing a person's right to practise is available to the Committee.

What happens once a complaint alleging misconduct is made?

(3.11) The practitioner's name is identified on the Council's register and then an officer of the Council will take action to assemble evidence available in support of the complaint.

(3.12) When the practitioner has been convicted in a criminal court, the conviction forms the basis (in most cases) on which the case will proceed. Further investigation is not required to establish the facts.

(3.13) In either case the practitioner is asked for a written statement, explanation or comment.

Preliminary Proceedings Committee procedures

Section 4

(4.1) The Preliminary Proceedings Committee considers cases which arise from convictions in Criminal Courts, reports received from public bodies such as Health Authorities/Boards, Trusts and complaints made by private individuals or professional colleagues.

(4.2) The Preliminary Proceedings Committee's powers are to determine whether, following a complaint made against a practitioner, the case of that practitioner should be:

(4.2.1) closed;
(4.2.2) referred to a Professional Conduct Committee for hearing;
(4.2.3) referred to the Panel of Professional Screeners, with a view to a hearing before the Health Committee; or
(4.2.4) closed by a formal caution as to future conduct.

(4.3) The Committee may also consider whether to impose interim suspension of a practitioner's registration, pending further investigation, and/or early referral to the Professional Conduct or Health Committee. This power will only be used, very occasionally, in circumstances where it is clear that in the interests of public safety, or in the practitioner's own interest, interim suspension should be imposed.

(4.4) The Preliminary Proceedings Committee will not normally meet the practitioner whose case is to be considered and will be making their judgement based upon written reports and evidence. The only exception will be when a Preliminary Proceedings Committee is considering imposing interim suspension, when the practitioner will have the right of audience and representation before the Committee. In these circumstances a special Committee of three Members of the Preliminary Proceedings Committee will be called to consider the case.

Professional Conduct Committee procedures

Section 5

(5.1) The points made in paragraph 2.3 again apply.

(5.2) The role of the Professional Conduct Committee is to consider cases of alleged misconduct which have been referred to it by the Preliminary Proceedings Committee.

(5.3) The Committee also considers applications for restoration to the register from persons whose names have previously been removed.

(5.4) The Professional Conduct Committee will have in attendance a legal assessor (to advise on admissibility of evidence and points of law) and a Council officer to advise on the Council's procedures and relevant background of the case. Respondents will normally be in attendance (but are not required to) at the professional conduct hearing and may be represented. The hearing is held in public.

(5.5) When considering allegations of misconduct or convictions arising from the Criminal Courts, the Professional Conduct Committee has the power to:

(5.5.1) find the practitioner not guilty of the matters alleged or, where the facts are proved, of misconduct and therefore close the case;
(5.5.2) take no further action on the misconduct it has proven and therefore close the case;
(5.5.3) issue a formal caution as to future conduct which will remain on the record for five years and may be used as antecedent history in the event of further misconduct and therefore close the case;
(5.5.4) postpone judgement, for a period it determines, on the misconduct it has proven;
(5.5.5) remove the practitioner's name from the register without a time limit or for a specified period;
(5.5.6) refer the practitioner's case to the Panel of Professional Screeners with a view to a hearing before the Health Committee; or
(5.5.7) impose interim suspension of the practitioner's registration, if the hearing is adjourned and it is considered necessary in the interest of the practitioner or public protection to do so.

(5.6) The purpose of the hearing is to concentrate on the matters which feature in the charges formally notified to the practitioner and is not to elicit evidence of other unsatisfactory behaviour.
(5.7) It is essential that the incident, if proved to the standard set out in paragraph 2.1, is considered in the context of its occurrence rather than in isolation.
(5.8) Information about the previous history of the practitioner is extremely important. It sometimes emerges that the incident in question occurred when the pressure of work was severe, that the practitioner was immediately honest and open about it and that the previous record over many years was exemplary.
(5.9) If, during the course of a hearing, evidence of possible ill health of the practitioner becomes available, the Professional Conduct Committee can decide to refer a case for consideration by the Health Committee.

Types of offences which may lead to removal from the register

Section 6

(6.1) The Council's Annual Reports from 1984 to 1992 provide information about how often particular types of proven charges have featured in cases which resulted in removal from the register.
(6.2) Practice-related offences are always at or near the top of the list. These are offences which show a failure to honour the primacy of the interest of patients.
(6.3) Frequently occurring reasons for removal from the register are:

(6.3.1) reckless and wilfully unskilful practice;
(6.3.2) concealing untoward incidents;
(6.3.3) failure to keep essential records;
(6.3.4) falsifying records;

(6.3.5) failure to protect or promote the interest of patients/clients;
(6.3.6) failure to act knowing that a colleague or subordinate is improperly treating or abusing patients;
(6.3.7) physical or verbal abuse of patients/clients;
(6.3.8) abuse of patients by improperly withholding prescribed drugs, or administering unprescribed drugs or an excess of prescribed drugs;
(6.3.9) theft from patients or employers;
(6.3.10) drug related offences;
(6.3.11) sexual abuse of patients; and
(6.3.12) breach of confidentiality.

(6.4) These categories of offence are not the only ones which have resulted in removal. They are simply those which have been regarded as particularly reprehensible. No two cases are the same in their details or context.

Types of cases referred for Professional Conduct Committee hearings which have not culminated in removal

Section 7

(7.1) Attention has already been drawn to the required standards of evidence and proof. Where that standard is not satisfied, the allegations are not proven and the respondent practitioner is declared not guilty of misconduct.

(7.2) There are a significant number of cases in which the facts are established, but which are not seen as misconduct by the Professional Conduct Committee when considered in context. This decision concludes the case.

(7.3) Cases most often found in this category include:

(7.3.1) offences related to motor vehicles;
(7.3.2) issues that relate specifically to employment, such as leaving duty early without authority, overtime claims in excess of hours worked, or mistakes disclosed by the practitioner which were made under pressure of work;
(7.3.3) cases where the practitioner's failure was effectively a failure to achieve the impossible in the particular circumstances that applied;
(7.3.4) cases which result from careful and conscientious exercise of professional judgement by the practitioner and which can be justified as reasonable in the circumstances and at the time the decision was taken; and
(7.3.5) situations where the case has been brought by a complainant measuring the actions of the practitioner against outdated practices and norms.

(7.4) When the facts alleged and misconduct are proven, certain reasons may emerge which lead the Professional Conduct Committee to decide that the practitioner's name should not be removed from the register. These have included cases where:

(7.4.1) the incident was isolated and uncharacteristic and the practitioner appears to have learnt lessons from it;
(7.4.2) there were, at the time, overwhelming personal problems which led the practitioner to behave inappropriately and which have since been resolved;
(7.4.3) the practitioner has been retained in employment and is the subject of good reports;
(7.4.4) the practitioner, having been responsible for an error, has made no attempt to conceal it and has immediately reported it in the interests of the patient;
(7.4.5) with hindsight it is clear that the incident was an error in professional judgement rather than a culpable act;
(7.4.6) the practitioner was one of a number involved, but the only person to be the subject of complaint; and
(7.4.7) removal is judged to be too harsh a response to the facts that have been established.

(7.5) In addition to the above, there have been rare occasions where the incidents have occurred in a stressful work setting with highly dependent patients, poor staffing and limited resources. Senior managers appear to have been fully aware of the deficiencies of the work environment but have taken no effective remedial action. In these circumstances, and in those particular cases heard by the Professional Conduct Committee, it was believed that removal of the name of the practitioner would be an inappropriate response to the problem.

Complaints alleging unfitness to practise due to illness

Section 8

Who can express concern that a practitioner may be unfit to practise due to illness?

(8.1) As with misconduct, anyone can express concern and initiate the process through which a practitioner's possible unfitness due to illness will be assessed and a decision made about her registration status. Such an expression of concern should be made to the Council.

(8.2) The Preliminary Proceedings Committee or Professional Conduct Committee can refer a case which has been brought to its attention as an allegation of misconduct.

When should concern that a practitioner's fitness to practise is impaired be expressed to the Council?

(8.3) Where such concerns emerge in the course of Preliminary Proceedings Committee or Professional Conduct Committee consideration of a case, and become a matter of formal record, the case is transferred immediately for assembly of medical evidence.

(8.4) In all other cases, a person who becomes concerned about a practitioner's illness or disability should formally express this concern as soon as she is satisfied that it appears to have seriouly impaired the ability to practise safely, provided the illness leading to impairment is not of a short-term nature. This action should not be seen as an alternative to offering local assistance to a practitioner who appears to be unwell.

How should these concerns be brought to the attention of the Council?

(8.5) A letter which provides brief details of the known illness or symptomatic behaviour giving rise to concern, together with sufficient information to identify the practitioner, should be sent to the Council. This category of case is known as a direct referral.

(8.6) Where possible, copies of any documents providing further information about the alleged unfitness to practise should be enclosed with the letter.

(8.7) Using the letter and enclosures from the person making the referral, the Council's solicitor draws up a statutory declaration for that person to sign. This document is a requirement of the law; without it an investigation of a practitioner's alleged unfitness to practise cannot proceed.

Professional Screeners' procedures

Section 9

(9.1) Once the statutory declaration has been signed and returned to the Council, the case is formally opened and considered by a group of Council Members (the Panel of Screeners) who look at documentary evidence and decide whether it should be pursued or closed. If it is to be pursued, the Screeners then decide on the category of specialist medical examiners to whom they wish the practitioner to be referred.

(9.2) On receipt of the medical examiners' reports, the Screeners then decide whether the practitioner's case should be referred to the Health Committee, referred back to the Preliminary Proceedings Committee or Professional Conduct Committee if that was the source of referral or closed.

By whom are the medical examinations conducted?

(9.3) The Council is required to maintain a panel of medical examiners covering a wide range of specialities. These examiners are appointed after nomination by specialist bodies such as the Royal Colleges of Physicians and Psychiatrists.

(9.4) Whenever possible, practitioners are referred to examiners who are geographically convenient. The medical examiners, however, will never be persons who practise in the same area as the referred practitioner. The full cost of examinations and travel is met by the Council.

Does the practitioner have access to the medical reports?

(9.5) Yes. As soon as reports are received by Council's staff, they are copied and sent to the practitioner, who then has a period of time to decide whether to choose a medical practitioner from whom to commission additional reports.

Health Committee procedures

Section 10

(10.1) Because of the nature of the material to be considered, the hearing is conducted in private. The Health Committee for each case is composed of five Council Members supported by an officer and a legal assessor. One of the medical examiners, whose reports form an essential part of the material before the Committee, must be present. The practitioner is encouraged to attend and may require that both examiners attend. She can be represented by a person or organisation of her choice and may also bring medical advisers and relatives or friends.

(10.2) In the majority of cases the practitioner accepts the general accuracy and conclusions of the medical reports and allows them, together with any other medical reports commissioned, to form the basis of discussion about the contention that fitness to practise may be seriously impaired by illness.

(10.3) On very rare occasions the practitioner refuses the invitation to medical examination by the Council's selected examiners and exercises the right to have the persons making the allegations, together with other witnesses to the behaviour on which the allegation is based, called to give evidence under oath. In such a case, one or more of the medical practitioners drawn from the Council's panel of examiners will attend in the role of medical assessor to advise the Committee.

(10.4) The Health Committee is not constituted to decide whether allegations against, or expressions of concern for practitioners are proven, but rather to consider the medical evidence and to determine whether the practitioner's fitness to practise is seriously impaired by illness or not, and if so, whether the practitioner is likely to be a danger to the public. The practitioner is normally present (but is not required to) and may be represented.

(10.5) The powers available to the Health Committee are to:

(10.5.1) close the case if the Committee is of the opinion that the practitioner's fitness to practise is not seriously impaired by reason of ill health;

(10.5.2) refer the case back to the Preliminary Proceedings Committee or Professional Conduct Committee if that was the source of referral;

(10.5.3) suspend the practitioner's registration;

(10.5.4) remove the practitioner's name from the register whether or not for a specified period;

(10.5.5) postpone judgement; or

(10.5.6) impose interim suspension of the practitioner's registration, if the hearing is adjourned and it is considered necessary in the interest of public safety or the practitioner's own interest to do so.

Types of illness which may culminate in removal from the register

Section 11

(11.1) Each case is the subject of detailed consideration and any illness that results in serious impairment of fitness to practise can result in removal.

(11.2) Conditions which have featured most frequently where practitioners' names have been removed from the register have been:

(11.2.1) alcohol dependence;
(11.2.2) other drug dependence; and
(11.2.3) various forms of mental illness.

Summary and conclusion

Section 12

(12.1) This document should not be read as an attempt to deter potential complainants from seeking investigation and judgement of those actions or omissions of practitioners which cause them particular concern, nor should it be read as an attempt to deter the reporting of ill practitioners in whose hands patients and clients may be at risk. On the contrary, by providing information about the system, the standards that must be satisfied and the outcome of cases in the recent past, it seeks to make sure that there is no delay to cases which need to be dealt with expeditiously in the interests of patients and clients.

(12.2) The potential complainant, before making a complaint, must consider whether the outcome she is seeking is for the practitioner's registration to be suspended or removed. If this is not the outcome the complainant is seeking, she should think carefully and consider seeking advice before submitting the complaint.

(12.3) Persons considering forwarding complaints alleging misconduct should ask themselves whether they personally consider the matter to be misconduct in a professional sense before formally making a complaint against a named individual.

(12.4) It is wise to refer to the two items the Professional Conduct Committee Members will have in mind. The first of these is the definition of misconduct in the statutory rules which states that 'Misconduct is conduct unworthy of a registered nurse, midwife or health visitor'. The second is the 'Code of Professional Conduct' for the Nurse, Midwife and Health Visitor, a copy of which is available from the Distribution Room at the Council.

(12.5) If the potential complainant takes the view that the matter (if proved to the required standard) is misconduct, she ought to go further and consider whether it raises a question only about the practitioner's appropriateness to continue in her present post or, alternatively, raises serious questions about her appropriateness to practise with patients/clients. If the conclusion is that it falls into the latter category, it should be forwarded. If it is the former, there may be little point in forwarding the complaint. Only the potential complainant can make this decision.

(12.6) If the potential complainant takes the view that a particular practitioner is ill, she needs to consider carefully whether the illness seriouly impairs the practitioner's fitness to practise.

(12.7) Questions arising from this advisory paper should be directed to the:

Assistant Registrar, Professional Conduct
United Kingdom Central Council
for Nursing, Midwifery and Health Visiting
23 Portland Place
London
W1N 3AF

Annexe A
A simplified illustration of the process by which an allegation of misconduct is considered by the Preliminary Proceedings Committee

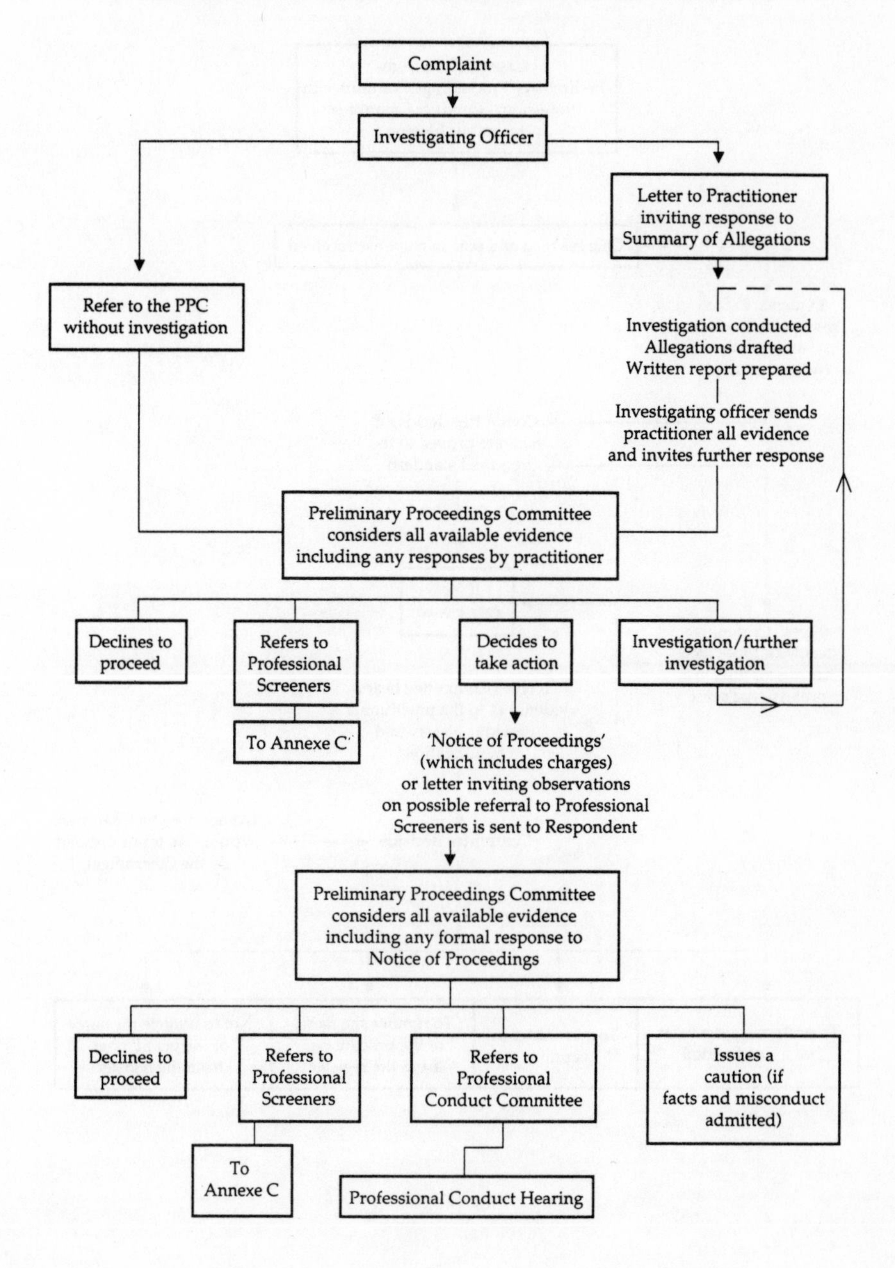

Annexe B
A simplified illustration of the process by which an allegation of misconduct is considered by the Professional Conduct Committee

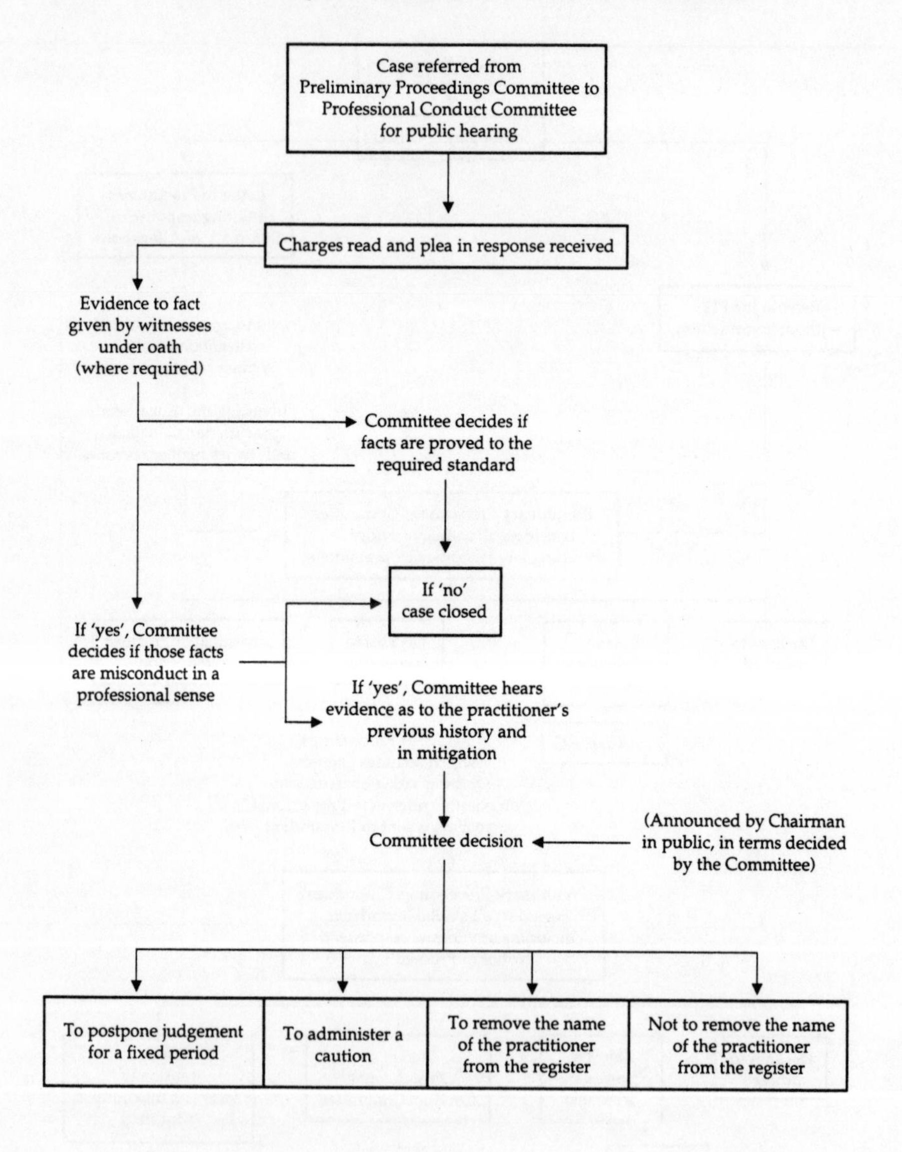

Annexe C

A simplified illustration of the process by which complaints alleging unfitness to practise are considered

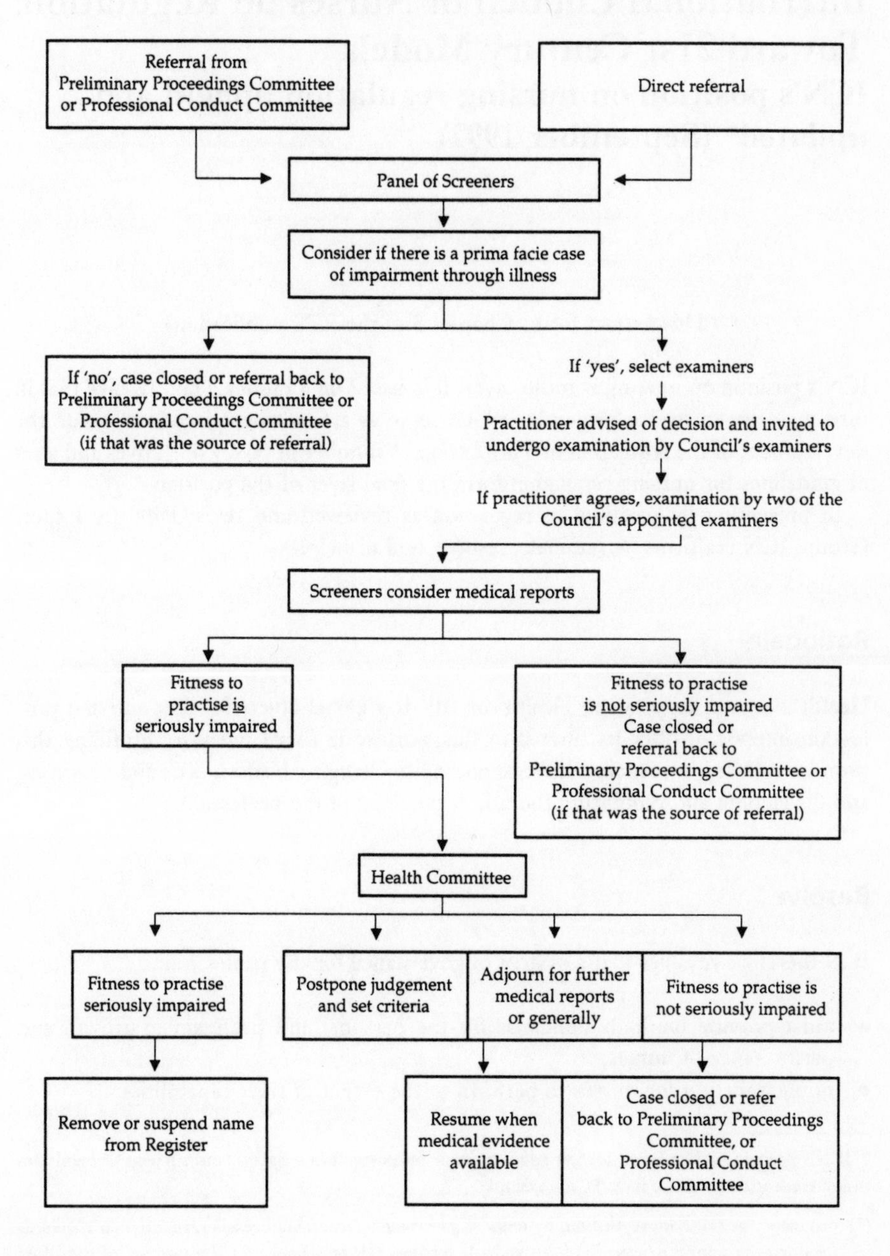

Appendix 7

International Council of Nurses on Regulation: Toward 21st Century Models

ICN's position on nursing regulation upheld and updated* (September 1997)

(This extract forms Chapter 3 of the ICN publication)

ICN's position on nursing is multi-layer. It is based on a rationale and resolve that in turn give rise to twelve principles which serve as a fundamental code to guide the development of the regulation of a profession. A number of policy objectives and a set of guidelines for nursing regulation form the final layer of the position.

In presenting its position on regulation as reviewed and revised by the Expert Group, ICN reaffirms its rationale, resolve, and principles.

Rationale

Health is a vital social asset; Health for All[1] is a global objective. The nursing profession intends to offer its utmost to this worldwide social purpose. Fulfilling this promise calls for influencing and responding to changing health needs and priorities; and developing and mobilising the fullest potential of the profession.

Resolve

ICN therefore resolves that a system of governance for the profession:

- must provide for high standards for the personal and professional growth and performance of nurses;
- public sanction for nurses to perform to the extent of their capabilities;

---

* ICN's position on regulation acknowledges multiple purposes, forms, agents, and subjects of regulation and credentialing. These include, for example:

(1) mandatory or statutory regulation, by units of government, enforcing licensing/registration standards for nurses or approval/accreditation standards for hospitals or schools, for the purpose of consumer protection;

(2) voluntary certification of nurse specialists or advanced practice nurses or accreditation of nursing schools or educational programmes, hospitals and other health services or products, by professional organisations or private agencies, for the purpose of designating particular competencies or standards of performance.

- participation of the profession in the development of public policy; accountability of the profession to the public for the conduct of its capabilities;
- participation of the profession in the development of public policy; accountability of the profession to the public for the conduct of its affairs in their behalf; and
- proper recognition and remuneration for the contributions of the profession and opportunity for the self-actualisation of its members.

Principles

I. Principle of purposefulness

Regulation should be directed toward an explicit purpose.

II. Principle of relevance

Regulation should be designed to achieve the stated purpose.

III. Principle of definition

Regulatory standards should be based upon clear definitions of professional scope and accountability.

IV. Principle of professional ultimacy

Regulatory definitions and standards should promote the fullest development of the profession commensurate with its potential social contribution.

V. Principle of multiple interests and responsibilities

Regulatory systems should recognise and properly incorporate the legitimate roles and responsibilities of interested parties – public, profession, government, employers, other professions – in aspects of standard-setting and administration.

VI. Principle of representational balance

The design of the regulatory system should acknowledge and appropriately balance interdependent interests.

VII. Principle of optimacy

Regulatory systems should provide and be limited to those controls and restrictions necessary to achieve their objectives.

VIII. Principle of flexibility

Standards and processes of regulation should be sufficiently broad and flexible to achieve their objectives and at the same time permit freedom for innovation, growth, and change.

IX. Principle of efficiency and congruence

Regulatory systems should operate in the most efficient manner, ensuring coherence and co-ordination among their parts.

X. Principle of universality

Regulatory systems should promote universal standards of performance and foster professional identity and mobility to the fullest extent compatible with local needs and circumstances.

XI. Principle of fairness

Regulatory processes should provide honest and just treatment for those parties regulated.

XII. Principle of interprofessional equality and compatibility

In standards and processes regulatory systems should recognise the equality and interdependence of professions.

Policy objectives for nursing regulation

The changes in the socio-political, economic and healthcare environment discussed in the previous chapter led the expert group to recommend a number of policy changes. Some of the modifications strengthen the original policy, some are additions, and others give a fresh emphasis to existing policies.

I. Principle of purposefulness

Regulation should be directed toward an explicit purpose.

Policy objectives for nursing

The overriding purpose of the statutory regulation of nursing is that of service to and protection of the public. Within the limits of its resources and authority, nursing needs to do its utmost to honour this intent and make available nursing care that is competent, accessible, effective and appropriate. This can only be achieved if:

(1) the organisation bearing the responsibility for regulating nursing is alert and innovative in fulfilling its role; and
(2) individual nurses adopt a dynamic approach to their role, striving to achieve their full potential in the service of the public and accepting responsibility to critically reappraise their practice as health care changes.

Benefits to the profession and individual practitioners are secondary and, although they can be significant, do not of themselves provide justification for statutory regulation. They may receive appropriate attention through other regulatory processes but the public interest must not be compromised as a result. It is appropriate and indeed desirable that the profession develop private or internal regulatory mechanisms to achieve other relevant goals, as, for example, recognition of competence in an advanced nursing field.

Such a dominant purpose has implications for the nursing profession and for the design and operation of a regulatory system that is imbedded in law. These are reflected in the subsequent principles and policy objectives.

II. Principle of relevance

Regulation should be designed to achieve the stated purpose.

Policy objectives for nursing

Since the overriding purpose of statutory regulation is service to and protection of the public, the regulatory system should be designed to satisfy this intent in a comprehensive manner.

Therefore, it is essential that:

(1) individual practitioners (a) recognise the importance of maintaining and improving their knowledge, skills, ethical awareness and competence throughout professional life; (b) use all opportunities to improve the quality and standard of nursing care, and (c) accept this responsibility as being an integral part of their personal accountability for professional practice; and
(2) practice settings are supportive of practitioners allowing practice to develop and flourish. To achieve this:
   - standards of education need to be relevant and be subjected to a regular review for continuing relevance;
   - examinations and other evaluation measures need to relate directly to these standards;
   - standards for practice and related performance reviews must be evaluated periodically to ensure they remain valid in changing circumstances; and
   - standards need to be relevant to the components of primary health care and strategies for achieving 'Health for All' and other societal goals. They must reflect broader health policy and be such that they have the potential to influence it.

III. Principle of definition

Regulatory standards should be based upon clear definitions of professional scope and accountability.

Policy objectives for nursing

A definition of *nursing* and *nurses* should be at the heart of every system for regulation of the profession.

The definitions should make it explicit that (a) the nurse is both responsible and accountable for the breadth of nursing practice, involving others where this is considered appropriate; and (b) there are circumstances in which the use of post-basic nurse specialists with knowledge and skill in a particular sphere of practice beyond that of the generalist nurse contributes maximally to providing the highest achievable quality of care.

Definitions of 'nurse' need to be clear and descriptive. They need also to communicate spheres of responsibility and accountability. Titles must convey a simple message as to who is the nurse, who is the nursing auxiliary (or support worker with another title), who is the specialist or advanced practice nurse in a particular area of practice.

ICN's clear preference, and therefore its strong recommendation, is that legislation adopt a flexible approach to 'scope of practice' issues. ICN recognises and accepts that benefits in service delivery can result from overlapping scopes of practice among different health professions and that a dynamic approach to professional practice will enable greater public service.

While recognising that at times such developments may be hampered by inappropriately restrictive professional legislation governing nursing or related health professions, ICN's position stems from an awareness of nursing's historic flexibility in adapting and expanding its role in response to changing and new health needs.

ICN, always mindful of the primacy of the public interest, provides a resource to assist the profession to develop and disseminate its views on core definitions, roles and the scope of practice.

IV. Principle of professional ultimacy

Regulatory definitions and standards should promote the fullest development of the profession commensurate with its potential social contribution.

Policy objectives for nursing

Since the function of a profession is, by definition, to serve society, nursing, in common with other health professions, should be encouraged to serve to its maximum capacity. As the complexities of health care and its social milieu increase, so must the capabilities of nurses, as citizens and practitioners, be heightened to meet new challenges.

To achieve this it is important that nurses, as individuals, as members of national nurses associations and, not least, as citizens of their countries, take every opportunity to influence events and contribute to policy debates which determine or affect the context of their professional practice. In this way they can become agents of constructive change for the public benefit and professional growth, rather than passive victims of potentially destructive change proposed and promoted by others.

National nurses associations should play their full part in this process, seeking always to promote open and positive debate and participate in the arena where health policy is developed.

Similar responsibility lies with the bodies authorised by statute to regulate the nursing profession. It cannot be regarded as acceptable that, through published codes, guidelines and standards documents, these bodies state their expectations of practitioners, but remain silent about the broader arena of health policy and the context in which nurses have to practise.

Advances in education for practice have a reciprocal relationship with innovations in practice and developments in research. Recognising this, and working within broad definitions that permit the profession's natural progression:

(1) educational programmes should encourage the development of nursing's potential through liberal, social, scientific and technical education;
(2) nursing service standards should reflect both changing needs and enhanced professional capacities; and
(3) the role of nursing research should be valued and reinforced.

V. Principle of multiple interests and responsibilities

Regulatory systems should recognise and incorporate the legitimate roles and responsibilities of interested parties – public, profession and its members, government, employers and other professions – in various aspects of standard-setting and administration.

Policy objectives for nursing

The profession

The profession's role in statutory regulation is very broad and of the greatest importance. For the profession (both through its national nurses' associations and the individual nurses of which it is composed) to fulfil this role satisfactorily, it must be vigilant in monitoring the operating effectiveness of existing regulatory arrangements and their sensitivity to the 'public interest'. Where the Government fails to provide consumer protection, the profession must be prepared to take the initiative and advance ideas and promote discussion that lead to constructive change of the regulatory system. It is not acceptable for the profession to be a passive participant always reacting to proposals from other sources.

It is the responsibility of the profession to take the leading role in its professional governance. This includes securing full participation of its members in statutory regulatory processes. As always these activities need to be sensitive to and respect the public interest. All this must be underpinned by an enhanced understanding among nurses of the purpose, processes and value of professional regulation.

The profession's role includes establishing and recommending the standards in the form of definitions, ethical codes, education and service requirements and a range of related issues. Further to this, the profession must bear the primary responsibility for development of the knowledge and skill base for all nursing, and for advancing nursing through fostering relevant post-basic specialist preparation and advanced nursing practice. This requires appropriate arrangements for credentialing, and research that enlarges the knowledge base for practice on a continuing basis.

To establish the profession's role in the regulation of practitioners and services, it is necessary that elements of this role be clearly acknowledged in government statutes, regulations or guidelines.

The profession also has a substantial part to play in the administrative aspects of governmental regulation, directly or by delegation. It can contribute its technical and interpretative expertise to nursing boards or councils and, while respecting the primacy of the public interest, continue to represent its own interests and those of its practitioners.

Most fundamentally, the profession, through its culture and ethic and its regulatory mechanisms, must promote the personal growth of its individual members. It must promote vigorously that component of professional regulation which the individual practitioner imposes *on herself or himself as a matter of personal professional accountability. Such self-regulation by nurses involves responsibility for developing their own capacities; participating in their own governance; and fulfilling their personal obligations to the people, practice, society, co-workers, and the profession as outlined in the ICN Code for Nurses.*[2] The profession, through the *national nurses' associations*, must provide a forum for discussing and achieving consensus regarding all critical matters of health care and professional governance. The collective capability to present conclusions knowledgeably, skilfully and concertedly in the public arena must be developed. It is through all these means – standard setting, participation in administrative aspects of governmental regulation, knowledge development and transmission, creating the culture and ethic for its members, and joining in public policy development – that the profession expresses its rights and related responsibilities and states its position on autonomy. *It is through acceptance of responsibilities in all of these areas that the profession makes its claim to and exercises self-governance.*

The Government

The Government's primary role in professional regulation for nursing should be to establish appropriate legislation. Statutory regulation needs to promote nursing's ability to respond to the societal needs and support nursing's role in primary health care services and in meeting the 'Health for All' objectives. The Government's supplementary role should be to administer, either directly or by delegation, a system to implement the law to regulate education, practice and the employment setting. Second, the Government's role is to protect the practitioner's right to title, practice, and compensation. Additionally, the Government, being responsible for public policy regarding health care priorities and resources, is obligated to guarantee nursing's access to policy development commensurate with its potential.

Related professions

Related professions have the right to participate in nursing's external governance processes to promote complementarity of the professions in the public interest. In this capacity their major roles are to provide liaison and technical advice. The nursing profession should expect reciprocal arrangements to exist. Moreover, all of the health professions have a right and responsibility to participate collaboratively in the formulation of health policies and priorities.

The employers

Employers, too, have an essential role to play in monitoring the standards for the profession for which, in the majority of cases, they provide the practice setting. In this capacity, with an awareness of the standards proposed and promoted by the professions, their principal role is to articulate their own institutional standards and nursing's part in meeting those standards. Furthermore, in serving society to the best of their ability, employers should provide an optimum milieu for achieving the maximum potential of nurse employees, an atmosphere in which they can fulfil their responsibility to comply with ethical and practice standards, and take appropriate action when they observe contravention of these standards.

Employers should recognise the benefits that stem from the individual professional registration or licensure as it provides the confirmation that a practitioner possessing a current licence has, in an initial and continuing sense, satisfied the requirements for such licensure and is accountable to the regulatory body that granted that licence. As appropriate, employers should also appreciate and utilise the credentials of nurse specialists and advance practice nurses within their practice and compensation structures.

Health care institutions and community-based services, like the professions, must submit to external review and public scrutiny, to ascertain that they are safe environments dedicated to the public interest, and that professional practice standards are observed and supported. Nurses who are self-employed or working in independent practice in partnership with professional colleagues have a responsibility to ensure that their working environment (for example, policies, physical resources, means of updating knowledge and skill) is adequate to support compliance with professional and service standards.

The public

Members of the public, where appropriate and possible and when it is consistent with a society's conventions, should be encouraged to participate in the regulatory processes. This helps to increase the visibility of the profession's collective accountability for its practice. Public representatives must understand their role and the healthcare and regulatory policies and systems. The primary role of the public representatives is to interpret and represent the public's needs and wishes and to collaborate with others in monitoring the content, application and consistency of standards and procedures forming part of the regulatory system. They should be invited to join health professionals to participate in public policy development to ensure that the essential purpose of the health care system and role of health professions are observed. It is incumbent on the profession to find creative ways for genuine public involvement in debate on regulatory and health policy.

VI. Principle of representational balance

The design of the regulatory system should acknowledge and appropriately balance interdependent interests.

Policy objectives for nursing

The important leading role which nurses, either individually or collectively, should play in the regulation of their profession has been emphasised in the policy objectives arising out of principle V. The role of other parties in the process has also been identified.

As the role and responsibility of the various legitimate interests are implemented through the participation of those who represent such interests in the various functions of the regulatory system, the reason for their participation and the principal purpose of regulation should be explicit. It is not in the best interest of the public for any profession to be unchallenged in its regulatory standards and processes. The profession may misunderstand or undervalue the public interest it purports to serve. Similarly, it is not in the public interest for any profession to dominate another, or to develop in disregard of the other professions to which it is linked in professional practice and with which it may share an overlapping scope of practice. By the same token, the regulatory processes must not be dominated by Government or its appointed participants.

Satisfactory health outcomes for the public will depend on good cooperation between the different health professions in regulation and practice. It is in the public interest that freedom for innovation and initiative in each of the health professions exists, and that service developments and choice in practice are not restricted.

Furthermore, it is to the benefit of the public that multiple and sometimes competing interests be recognised, avoided and minimised, and dealt with within the regulatory system. For example, a potential conflict of interest exists when management and the accreditation of schools and services are vested within the same authority. This raises a potential conflict between measures to cut costs and efforts to set and maintain standards. In such cases, mechanisms to consider all viewpoints must be provided through some internal process or, more effectively, through an external review.

VII. Principle of professional optimacy

Regulatory systems should provide and be limited to those controls and restrictions necessary to achieve their objectives.

Policy objectives for nursing

The purpose of statutory regulation is to ensure that competent and accessible care is available from truly accountable practitioners and this should be done using efficient, effective and economic processes. *Governments*, in developing or revising arrangements for a sound statutory base for the regulation should concentrate on the best way to achieve this. Their focus should be on the mandatory credentialing and career-long monitoring of nurses.

Exclusive focus on controlling basic education and the screening of practitioners only on the first entry to practice is inadequate to ensure continuing competence. Failure to apply appropriate regulatory controls to the environment in which credentialed nurses practise falls short of a comprehensive regulatory programme. These three examples may represent circumstances of *too little regulation*.

Conversely, *over-regulation* – particularly where it limits opportunities for innovations in practice, imposes inappropriate scope of practice restrictions or fails to recognise the logic of overlapping scopes of practice between professions – is contrary to the public interest.

A failure by the authorised regulatory body to offer remedial or rehabilitation opportunities during the exercise of its powers of discipline may be seen as disregarding the *optimacy* principle. A regulatory body acting optimally has some means to assist nurses regain the ability and authority to practise, if it is still in the public interest.

Proposals to introduce some form of the state regulation of auxiliaries should recognise that auxiliaries should work under the direct or indirect supervision of nurses with whom the ultimate responsibility lies, and should not recommend arrangements that erode this principle. The supervision referred to may be the exercise of oversight or surveillance by a professional practitioner who has assessed the situation, identified the need for nursing intervention, determined the nature of that intervention and continues to retain accountability for the care given. It is recognised that employers, either individually or collectively, or through local or national voluntary accrediting schemes, might choose to encourage a level of regulation of this category of direct care employees.

While it is important to avoid over-regulation, it is equally important, in situations in which professional practitioners and auxiliaries constitute parts of the same service team, to ensure clarity of titles, roles, and responsibilities.

Nurses who qualify as *post-basic specialists* are, by virtue of their basic qualification, already the subject of regulation by the body authorised for this purpose. It is, however, appropriate for the basic registration to be supplemented to indicate that the nurse is a specialist in a particular area of practice, by virtue of additional education and demonstrated competence. This holds true for advanced practice nurses, as well.

An optimum system is, therefore, likely to incorporate:

(1) approval and, thereafter, periodic accreditation of schools which prepare nurses for licensure;
(2) initial credentialing and, thereafter, periodic licensure (subject to certain criteria being satisfied) for individual practitioners;
(3) supplementary entries in addition to those of basic licensure to indicate areas of specialist status and advanced practice;
(4) standards, criteria and related support and monitoring systems for health service settings; and
(5) appropriate disciplinary procedures and sanctions for practitioners and practice settings.

Whatever the system, the principle of *optimacy* should be carefully observed and the purpose of regulation honoured.

VIII. Principle of flexibility

Standards and processes of regulation should be sufficiently broad and flexible to achieve their objective and at the same time permit freedom for innovation, growth and change.

Policy objectives for nursing

Just as governmental regulation should be neither too little nor too much, it should be neither too general nor too specific. In particular, scope of practice definitions and associated educational standards should give broad guidance to practitioners and employers through general statements of nursing function. Similarly, broad guidance to schools on required subject areas, faculty specifications and learning resource requirements is to be preferred over detailed prescription of procedures and curriculum content. To maintain relevance as practice changes and achieve ultimacy as the profession seeks to reach its potential, flexibility is essential in supporting the development and exercise of professional judgement skills and the search for creative solutions to practice situations.

Additionally the mobility of the practitioner may be compromised if the authority to practise is granted at an institutional level and limited to that institution's mandate. Though not without validity in some circumstances, it cannot have the same public credibility emanating from individual licensure granted by a statutory body for practice in a province, state or country.

IX. Principle of efficiency and congruence

Regulatory systems should operate in the most efficient manner, ensuring coherence and coordination among their parts.

Policy objectives for nursing

Regulatory activity on the part of and between (a) levels of Government, (b) categories of personnel, (c) related professions and (d) education and practice should be coordinated to accomplish the purpose of regulation in a uniform streamlined fashion. The design of the system should incorporate structural arrangements appropriate to the local circumstances. For example, such means include single statutes, single authorities, centralised and consolidated agencies, cross-participation in credentialing, and liaison activities, provided they contribute to the basic purpose in an effective and efficient way and do not compromise interested parties. It is essential that, whatever the arrangements, they involve opportunity for cross-disciplinary consultation. These same arrangements apply, in a general way, to the interface between statutory and private or voluntary regulatory mechanisms that exist within the profession.

X. Principle of universality

Regulatory systems should promote universal standards of performance and foster professional identity and mobility to the fullest extent compatible with local needs and circumstances.

Policy objectives for nursing

Although some adaptation to local circumstances is desirable, and accepting the need to be sensitive to cultural differences in developing regulatory procedures, it should be recognised that wide divergence may lead to instability in the workforce and variable standards of care. Substantial inconsistency is also antithetical to the achievement of broad and uniform development of the profession and the free movement of practitioners. While jurisdictions may adopt temporary measures to accommodate existing conditions, the international goal of 'Health for All' and the principle of *professional ultimacy* mandate that standards of education and practice commensurate with increasing rigour of health care requirements (and relevant to the local needs) be set by nations as a long-range plan. International trade agreements and the globalisation movements may create a climate and need for international credentials with worldwide acceptance, giving new meaning to the *universality* principle.

Countries should look to the ICN and the WHO for guidance in setting and achieving standards and in developing strategies for change.

XI. Principle of fairness

Regulatory processes should provide honest and just treatment for those parties regulated.

Policy objectives for nursing

The features of an honest and just system of regulation, whether it deals with practitioners, schools, or service agencies are:

(1) relevant standards and procedures;
(2) provide full information regarding criteria and processes;
(3) encourage open discussion and comprehensive policy debate involving all those who will be affected;
(4) use objective measurement and review;
(5) give ample opportunity to appeal decisions; and
(6) provide fair treatment for complainants including reasonable access and the right of appeal against decisions.

These features should be incorporated in the design of the regulatory system and should lead to greater satisfaction of all involved parties. However, they must not jeopardise the public interest, which is the prime purpose of regulation.

Application of the principle of *fairness* will also mean that practitioners honouring their obligations as stated in the ICN Code for Nurses[2] and their respective national codes and acting out of conviction can expose actions or omissions (whether on the part of individuals or institutions) that are against the public interest, without fear of recrimination.

During periods of transition for the profession, when standards are being raised or augmented, practising nurses should be provided protection of their credentials and/or opportunity for improving their qualifications.

The introduction of more uniform standards and procedures, based on a dynamic standard-setting approach and applied research, and shared across national, state and provincial boundaries has the potential to facilitate the mobility of nurses, provided that national regulatory laws are not unnecessarily restrictive. Multinational pacts have promoted such developments. However, where this applies, it is necessary to ensure that the freedom to move between a number of countries is founded on a common agreement governing education and training leading to the granting of licensure that is honestly applied by all involved. Both types of development can help to promote a singular, international identification for nurses and nursing.

XII. Principle of interprofessional equality and compatibility.

In standards and processes, regulatory systems should recognise the equality and interdependence of professions offering essential services.

Policy objectives for nursing

For professions to develop and to work collaboratively on the public behalf, education and practice standards need to be comparable and regulatory processes complementary. Nursing must be central to the professional mainstream and should position itself at the heart of debates and policy-making with respect of these matters.

Nursing should aim to fit within the dominant education and regulatory pattern in each country. Education for nursing should occur in the same setting, at the approximate level, and with similar autonomy as for other professions. Statutory regulation of nurses should parallel that of other professions. If it is customary for physicians and other health professionals to serve on regulatory boards for nursing in prescribed numbers, the reverse is equally fitting. Furthermore, nursing should not be treated differently from other professions with respect to the incorporation of information concerning personal status and qualifications in the regulatory body's records which are available to public and employers. In summary, in order to participate as a full and responsible partner in the health care team, nursing should closely associate with and be on a par with other professions and be dealt with similarly in regulatory policies and practices.

It does not, however, stop there. As the largest of the regulated health professions, composed of the practitioners who spend the greatest amount of time in direct contact with members of the public requiring health services, nursing must accept the responsibility to take the lead in monitoring existing regulatory arrangements; in generating ideas and promoting debate leading to positive change in those arrangements; and in introducing improvements in regulatory standards and processes. These are ways of demonstrating the profession's awareness of the primacy of the public interest and total commitment to serving that interest.

The above principles and policy objectives for nursing regulation, first introduced in 1985, have been upheld and updated in workshops throughout the world between 1988 and 1992 and most recently by the deliberations of the Expert Group. They continue to serve as the foundation for the twenty-first century model.

References

1. *Renewing the Health-for-All Strategy. Elaboration of a Policy for Equity, Solidarity and Health* (1995). Consultation Document. Geneva: World Health Organization.
2. *Code for Nurses* (1973) (Reaffirmed in 1989). Geneva: International Council of Nurses.

Table of Cases

Chapter 13

Chapter 14

Recommended Reading

Beardshaw, V. (1981) *Conscientious Objectors at Work*. Social Audit Limited, London.

Brykcznska, G. (ed.) (1989) *Ethics in Paediatric Nursing*. Chapman and Hall, London.

Burnard, P. & Chapman, C. (1988) *Professional and Ethical Issues in Nursing*. John Wiley, Chichester/New York.

Chadwick, R. & Tadd, W. (1992) *Ethics and Nursing Practice: A case study approach*. Macmillan Education, London.

Dimond, B. (1993) *Patients' Rights, Responsibilities and the Nurse*. Quay Publishing, Lancaster.

Dimond, B. (1995) *Legal Aspects of Nursing*. Prentice Hall, London.

Dyer, C. (ed.) (1992) *Doctors, Patients and the Law*. Blackwell Science, Oxford.

Fry, S.T. (1994) *Ethics in Nursing Practice: A Guide to Ethical Decision Making*. International Council of Nurses, Geneva.

Heywood Jones, I. (1990) *The Nurse's Code*. Macmillan Education, London.

Johnstone, M-J. (1994) *Bioethics: a nursing perspective*. W.B. Saunders, Sydney.

Melia, K. (1989) *Everyday Nursing Ethics*. Macmillan Education, London.

Rowson, R. (1990) *An Introduction to Ethics for Nurses*. Scutari Press, London.

Rumbold, G. (1985) *Ethics in Nursing Practice*. Baillière Tindall, Eastbourne.

Stacey, M. (1992) *Regulating British Medicine*. John Wiley, Chichester/New York.

Tingle, J. & Cribb, A. (eds) (1995) *Nursing Law and Ethics*. Blackwell Science, Oxford.

Tschudin, V. (ed.) (1994) *Ethics: Conflict of Interest*. Scutari Press, London.

Index